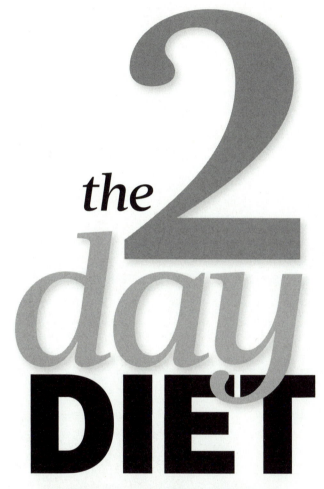

the 2 day DIET

PART-TIME DIET—
FULL-TIME RESULTS!

Sarí Harrar and the Editors of **Prevention**®

RODALE®

© 2013 by Rodale Inc.

Photographs © 2013 by Rodale Inc.

Printed in the United States of America

Rodale Inc. makes every effort to use acid-free ♾, recycled paper ♻.

Photographs by Mitch Mandel/Rodale Images

Book design by Christina Gaugler

Library of Congress Cataloging-in-Publication Data is on file with the publisher.

ISBN 978–1–60961–485–0 direct hardcover

4   6   8   10   9   7   5   3   hardcover

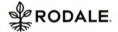

We inspire and enable people to improve their lives and the world around them.
For more of our products, visit prevention.com or call 800–848–4735.

With gratitude to all the members of our 2-Day Diet test panel.

Thanks for coming along on this exciting journey. Your success will

inspire others to live healthier, more active lives.

CONTENTS

PART I

The Power of

Wherever you are right now—standing in a bookstore, sitting at your kitchen table with a mug of coffee, or reading in the car while you wait to pick up the kids—we know you've got two burning questions you'd love to ask us about the 2-Day Diet:

Could something this simple really help me lose weight?

Can you prove it?

We asked ourselves the same things—and you'll find all the answers ahead in Part 1.

In Chapter 1, you'll discover the results of the 7-week test panel that proved to us just how amazing this plan is. We tracked 18 brave and generous individuals (16 women and 2 men), ranging in age from their twenties through their sixties, who test-drove the plan. You'll learn all of their nitty-gritty "before" and "after" details—including how much weight, how much body fat, and how many inches they lost. You'll read about their health improvements and about unexpected benefits such as brighter moods and deeper sleep.

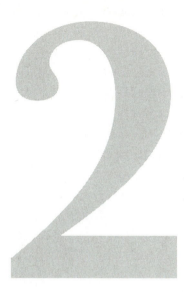

But how does it work? In Chapter 2, you'll delve into the provocative new science of low-carb eating for weight loss and weight maintenance—as well as the fascinating, research-backed realm of part-time dieting. Our cutting-edge plan combines these two approaches, maximizing the benefits while minimizing the downsides. Got health concerns? You've come to the right place. In Chapter 3, you'll discover tantalizing evidence about the power of this approach to lower risk for major health threats such as diabetes, heart disease, and even some forms of cancer.

Our 2-Day Diet Workout gets its own "how it works" chapter, as well. In Chapter 4, we outline why devoting just 2 days a week to easy, superefficient interval training and strength training (toning) torches calories and fat while giving your muscles a youthful makeover.

If we could give Part I a subtitle, it would be "Yes, It Works, and Here's Why." We know you'll come away impressed, inspired, and ready to start your own 2-Day Diet journey.

CHAPTER 1

The 2-Day Diet:
Easiest Weight
Loss Ever!

It's a dieter's dream come true. Diet just 2 days a week and lose *more* pounds, *more* inches, *more* body fat, and *more* belly fat than you would on a conventional pounds-off plan[1]—without feeling hungry, deprived, bored, or worried that your next little slipup could throw all your hard work out the window. That's the promise of the 2-Day Diet, the breakthrough weight-loss plan proven to help you slim down, tone up, and feel great. Yes, just 2 days a week. It couldn't be simpler.

■ **Follow our delicious, dietitian-designed, low-carb eating plan just *2 days a week,* then eat normal portions of healthy foods on our "regular-carb" plan the other 5**. You'll enjoy satisfying, tastebud-tickling meals such as Coconut-Almond Pancakes and bacon and eggs for breakfast; hot turkey-and-cheese sandwiches and roast beef and guacamole for lunch; and Walnut-Crusted Chicken Breasts with Basil Sauce and Taco Burgers with Tex-Mex Salad for dinner. Help yourself to a daily snack, too, like a Chocolate-Almond Smoothie or a Strawberry Cream Frostie (so delicious that one of our test panelists is still making them for her family!), frozen yogurt, chocolate, walnuts, or Deviled Eggs with Hummus. Yum!

While you enjoy these flavorful, filling meals, this low-carb plan is busy turbocharging your body's ability to burn calories and torch fat. Then regular-carb days give you an all-important diet break proven to help you stay on track.

■ **Get active with our exclusive 2-Day Diet Workout.** No time? No problem. Get the results you want in the time you have with our superefficient, multitasking exercise plan. In just 2 days a week, this program blasts more body fat and burns more calories than old-fashioned steady-paced exercise routines. Designed by a fitness expert, this activity routine is based on the new science of interval training—alternating bouts of higher-paced and slower-paced activities shown to blast more fat and contribute to greater weight loss. Do the 2-Day Diet Workout interval routines for just 30 minutes twice a week as you walk or ride your exercise bike or even while you march, jog in place, or do calisthenics in front of the TV. Then add 10 to 15 minutes of strength-training, toning moves twice a week. Five simple exercises target all your major muscle groups, so you build sleek, shapely, calorie-blasting muscle all over in minutes flat.

Then watch as the pounds, inches, and body fat melt away—and the compliments roll in. Easy!

REAL-WORLD SUCCESS

The 2-Day Diet works. When 18 women and men test-drove the plan for 7 weeks, *everyone* lost body fat and inches and reduced their body mass index (BMI), a measure that compares weight to height. Among them: Renee Guzenski, 40, who dropped 15.8 pounds and trimmed 13.25 inches—including 4 inches from her hips and 2 inches from her waist. She did it while enjoying sirloin burgers, steak with blue cheese dressing, and hot turkey-and-cheese sandwiches for lunch. "I'm wearing clothes I couldn't get into before," says Renee, an accounting associate and mother of two.

Test panelist Paula Weiant, age 50, lost 9.2 pounds while working two jobs, being a mom to her 18-year-old daughter, taking care of the family dog (a pug mix named Olive), and still finding time to have a social life. (Yay, Paula!) She trimmed 3 inches from her waist and 3.75 inches from her hips—even though she took 1 night a week off to go out to eat with friends. She calls the plan "so user-friendly that you can't mess up."

Dale Honig, 67, lost 12.8 pounds during the 6-week plan—and went on to lose a total of 20 pounds when she stayed on the 2-Day Diet for 15 weeks. "Thanks again for sharing the 2-Day Diet plan," she e-mailed us 2 months after the official test panel ended in the summer of 2012. "It is making a difference in my life!"

It works for guys, too. Twenty-four-year-old Matt Opatovsky lost 20.8 pounds, including 18.2 pounds of body fat. Matt says that he's learned a lot about food and that it's changed the way he eats for the better. His breakfasts are a healthy mix of eggs and veggies, for example, and he's curtailed his morning stops for large, sugary coffee drinks. And test panelist Luis Rosario, 45, lost 14.8 pounds. He made over his body for the better, losing 21 pounds of body fat and building 6.2 pounds of lean, strong muscle. Luis also trimmed 3 inches from his waist and another 3 from his hips. Wow!

ZAP POUNDS, INCHES, AND BODY FAT—LIKE MAGIC

When a registered dietitian and fitness expert designed this plan for us, we were excited about its potential. But when our test panelists returned for their "after" weigh-ins, we were astounded by the results.

- **Average weight loss: 9.1 pounds.** Eight test panelists lost more than 11 pounds apiece—and four lost more than 15 pounds! *Together, our test panelists dropped a total of 164.2 pounds!*

- **Average body fat loss: 7.5 pounds.** Every test panelist shed body fat on the 2-Day Diet, with seven panelists losing 10 or more pounds of flab each! *Together, our test panelists said good-bye to a total of 135 pounds of fat!*

- **Average inches lost: 10.9.** All our test panelists lost inches—whittling their waistlines by an average of 3.6 inches, slimming their hips by 2.3 inches on average, and trimming their chest, upper arms, and thighs, too. Six test panelists dropped 4 or more inches from their waists. Two lost 9 or more inches. (Bye-bye, belly fat!) *Our test panelists trimmed a total of 196.2 inches!*

- **More muscle, less fat.** Thirteen panelists improved their muscle-to-fat ratio on the 2-Day Diet—including seven who built *more* lean muscle while losing weight. That's big news, because holding on to precious muscle mass can help you avoid weight-loss plateaus, make you look slimmer and trimmer, help you maintain your new lower weight in the long term, and even improve your health by lowering your risk for diabetes and heart disease. And as you'll discover later in this chapter, this amazing muscle benefit is something many weight-loss diets don't deliver—in fact, many secretly rob you of muscle, setting you up for trouble with the bathroom scale, with your clothes, with your figure, and even with your future health.

Great Health by the Numbers

"Before" and "after" checks prove it: Across the board, 2-Day Diet test panelists saw big improvements in their blood pressure, blood sugar, cholesterol, and triglyceride levels. Moving these important indicators into a healthier range can help lower the risk for diabetes, heart disease, and stroke. The exciting results:

◆ **Stellar blood sugar:** Seven test panelists saw their fasting blood sugar levels improve.

Average drop: 9.5 points

Biggest change: 14 points

◆ **Better blood pressure:** Eleven test panelists had lower blood pressure by the end of the 2-Day Diet.

Average drop: 13 points (systolic blood pressure (a measure of pressure during a heartbeat); 7 points diastolic blood pressure (a measure of pressure between heartbeats)

Biggest change: 32 points systolic, 16 points diastolic

◆ **Lower LDL cholesterol levels:** Thirteen test panelists saw reductions in their LDLs, the "bad" cholesterol that can clog artery walls and raise the risk for heart attacks and strokes.

Average drop: 17.5 points

Biggest change: 35 points

◆ **Trimmer triglycerides:** Levels of this heart-threatening blood fat fell for 11 test panelists.

Average drop: 47.8 points

Biggest change: 155 points

A REVOLUTION IN WEIGHT LOSS

Here at Rodale, we're dedicated to finding the newest, best, research-proven, and real-world-tested ways to help people like you make healthy changes that really last. So we were intrigued when we began hearing whispers about a brand-new approach to healthy weight loss being tested in a handful of forward-looking research labs in the United States and the United Kingdom. This new strategy combined the best of two tough yet effective pounds-off approaches—part-time dieting and low-carb dieting—while eliminating their downsides.

It was a marriage made in weight-loss heaven. For decades, scientists and physicians had experimented with part-time fasting to help extremely obese people lose large amounts of weight. As you'll discover in Chapter 2, this ultrasevere type of diet—some researchers called it "the starvation diet" or "the hunger diet"— certainly did erase pounds. *Lots and lots* of pounds. But fasting a few days every week isn't easy. Weight regain was common, and so were underlying side effects such as loss of muscle mass, which lowered metabolism and made weight maintenance even more difficult. The upside: major weight loss. The downside: nearly impossible to stick to.

Enter low-carb eating. Proven to help people lose plenty of weight, low-carb dieting caught the attention of British researchers looking for a way to help women at higher-than-average risk for breast cancer lose pounds and reverse body chemistry changes that boosted their vulnerability to cancer. The researchers wanted a plan that got big results in real-world conditions. They liked the idea of a part-time diet, but not fasting. At first, they experimented with ultra-low-calorie eating 2 days a week—and found that women lost weight and reduced levels of the hormones leptin and insulin, both of which can raise cancer risk. They also saw a drop in levels of inflammation-boosting proteins, which also lowers cancer risk. So far, so good. But living on 650 calories a day 2 days a week isn't easy. There had to be an even better way. They then experimented with low-carb

6 Weeks to a Slimmer, Sleeker You!

What kinds of results can you expect on the 2-Day Diet? Take a peek at the pounds, body fat, and inches our test panelists lost in just 6 weeks.

TOTAL POUNDS LOST: 164.2
Average weight loss: 9.1 pounds

Most weight lost: 20.8 pounds

The details: Ten test panelists lost more than 8 pounds. Of these "biggest losers," eight lost more than 11 pounds. And four of those shed more than 15 pounds!

TOTAL INCHES LOST: 196.2
Average all-over inches lost: 10.9—from the waist, chest, hips, upper arms, and thighs

Most inches lost: 21.25

The details: All test panelists lost inches—including an average of 3.6 inches from their waistlines and 2.3 inches from their hips. Two lost 9 or more inches from their waists; five lost 3 or more inches from their hips!

BODY FAT LOST: 135 POUNDS
Average body fat lost: 7.5 pounds

Most body fat lost: 21 pounds

The details: Every test panelist shed body fat. And seven panelists lost 10 or more pounds of fat each!

eating 2 days a week, letting study volunteers nosh on the healthy foods of their choice other days.

Bingo! This is when we really took notice. In a recent study, the women who followed a part-time low-carb plan lost more weight and saw bigger improvements in leptin, insulin, and inflammatory compounds than did women in a control group who followed a conventional reduced-calorie, full-time diet. Over 3 months, the low-carb group that cut out carbohydrate-packed foods like bread, breakfast cereal, noodles, crackers, and sweets just 2 days a week lost 9 pounds, while dieters who stuck with a 1,500-calorie plan every day lost just 5 pounds.

Amazing! Suddenly, full-time calorie counting seemed so old-fashioned. Watching carbs 2 days a week, it turns out, is more effective!

Inspired by their success, we developed the 2-Day Diet, a part-time, low-carb plan designed to fit into your busy life. We increased the daily carb count on low-carb days from the superlow 40 grams a day used in the British studies to a more generous, satisfying, and delicious 50 grams a day. That gave us "wiggle room" to include low-carb bread, fruit, and dairy products on low-carb days. And we created a regular-carb healthy-eating plan for the other 5 days of the week—a plan that relies on healthy portions of good food to keep you on track for weight-loss success, great health, and a lifetime of good eating.

Those 5 regular-carb days a week are essential. You get time off, which makes the 2-Day Diet so flexible that it's virtually fail-proof. Case in point: If you start a low-carb day and find you get off track, it's not a problem. Simply declare it a regular-carb day, then go low-carb another day! This plan is full of second chances—and third, fourth, fifth, sixth, and seventh chances. Since it's almost impossible to fall off the wagon, you'll never find yourself feeling you messed up, a common experience that spells disaster for full-time diets. Many test panelists told us that they loved the plan's flexibility precisely because it took the possibility of "failing" off the table. That breaks the diet mess-up cycle that leads to weight gain—you know, when you eat the "wrong" food, feel guilty, figure you've blown it, and have another bowl of ice cream. On this plan, if something gets in the way, you just start over tomorrow!

We also incorporated our own super-efficient workout program, designed by fitness expert Michele Stanten, former fitness director for *Prevention* magazine. In just two sessions a week, you'll burn calories, torch body fat, build fitness, and maintain or build muscle—all of which will help you lose weight, tone up, feel energized, and maintain your new, lower weight.

Put it all together and you've got the 2-Day Diet. You'll love the simplicity, the satisfaction, the small commitment of time, and the big-time results. And you'll feel great knowing this plan can also help you control your risk for major health threats such as diabetes, heart disease, brittle bones, cancer, and even memory and thinking problems. But that's not all. You'll also *feel* better than you have in years.

FEEL GREAT!

Over and over again, test panelists told us that they felt terrific thanks to the 2-Day Diet. They had more energy and brighter moods. They slept better. And they weren't the only ones to notice these positive changes. Friends, relatives, co-workers, and significant others saw the improvements, too. Throughout this book, you'll be reading about the experiences of our brave, adventurous, and generous test panelists. Look for special boxes marked "Test Panelist Tip" to learn more about how they dealt with all sorts of real-world challenges—from ordering with confidence in restaurants to making new foods taste great.

Even after their time on the diet, they continued to look and feel better and to see improvements in key health indicators.

"My boyfriend noticed it," says Kathy Rocchetti. "He was really glad I was doing the diet—not just for my body shape, but for my overall attitude. I was feeling good, not as moody, not so hyper. Now I'm happy and definitely not as stressed. I have more energy, and I'm sleeping better. My boyfriend is also doing the diet, and he's feeling happier, too."

Mary Banyas, who lost 11.2 pounds and 9.25 inches from her waistline, says she felt more energetic at what had historically been the low point of her day: midafternoon. "I used to depend on diet soda to get me through the afternoon, but I absolutely have more energy now," she says. "And when you're successful at losing weight, you just feel better about yourself. I'm slimmer. My skin even looks clearer. People at work have noticed a change in my outlook. I feel more positive!"

Michelle Sparr also got an energy upgrade. She deals with other people's computer problems all day long at work—and fields plenty of late-afternoon calls that require patience and creative problem solving. Her high-carb lunches used to leave her feeling physically and mentally drained late in the day. Now, she powers through the afternoon thanks to low-carb meals and no longer feels "draggy and tired and irritable."

THE MUSCLE ADVANTAGE

Did you know that conventional diets can "steal" lots of muscle while you're losing weight? You can't tell by looking at your bathroom scale whether the pounds

Attention, Moms and Dads: This Diet's Family Friendly!

Do you cook for the family or for yourself and your significant other? You'll be happy to hear that 2-Day Diet meals fit easily into family meals—no need to cook twice! Make the meals on the plan, then add an extra starch (a healthy one such as brown rice or a whole grain pasta) to please the crowd. That strategy worked for our test panelists, whose families enjoyed the hearty main dishes and sides on the plan.

- "My husband loved the sirloin burgers, the walnut-crusted chicken, and the steaks," says Sara Phillips. "He even lost 10 pounds!"

- Sharon Spitz, her husband, and their 4-year-old twins all skipped noodles and spaghetti while Sharon was on the plan. "We boycotted pasta," she says. "The kids liked the Taco Burgers and the Beef and Scallion Stir-Fry—even though they did pick the scallions out. We made it with chicken sometimes, too."

- Karen Fazioli found that a simple way to avoid cooking two different meals for the family was to cook up a 2-Day Diet meal, then serve extra vegetables, brown rice, or quinoa (another healthy grain) for her husband and three children. "It worked," she says. "I'm not a short-order cook—everyone eats the same meal in our household. The family really liked the 2-Day Diet main dishes like pork with fresh sauerkraut and the walnut-crusted chicken. I got rid of bread at most meals, but did make a grain side dish. Everybody was full and satisfied."

- Paula Weiant's 18-year-old daughter embraced the plan's healthy eating. "She's a dancer and doesn't need to lose weight, but she loved the meals because they were good for her and tasted good," says Paula. "She ate the turkey bacon at breakfast, loved the burgers and the chicken dishes, and still makes Chocolate-Almond Smoothies for breakfast."

- Michelle Sparr discovered she could convert some 2-Day Diet recipes into slow-cooker creations—saving time and giving her plenty of leftovers for another dinner or lunch. "My husband and stepdaughter really liked the pork dishes," she says. "I would make the pork picadillo from the 5-Day Jump Start in my slow cooker, using a pork loin. It turned out great!"

you've lost are flabby body fat or sleek, strong, calorie-burning muscle. But when Purdue University researchers checked the data from 52 diet studies, they found that up to half of the pounds that study volunteers lost on most diet programs were in fact precious muscle.[2]

That's a problem. Muscle is your body's "engine," burning calories all day and all night as it turns blood sugar and fatty acids into energy. Losing muscle lowers your metabolism, which sets you up for regain when you stop dieting. Muscle also keeps you strong, balanced, and healthy.

In contrast, the 2-Day Diet's revolutionary approach helps you hold on to more sleek, sexy, calorie-burning muscle as you lose weight—and even helps build more of this great stuff! You'll look slimmer, feel more energetic, and find that maintaining your new, lower weight is a breeze. How? This program pampers muscle three ways:

First, low-carb eating is proven to help you hold on to more muscle mass as you lose weight. Researchers call it "the metabolic advantage" of low-carb meals.[3]

Second, low-carb eating helps muscle cells stay more active. In one fascinating new study, successful dieters who were trying to maintain their new, lower weight were put on a low-carb diet, a low-fat diet, or a balanced low-glycemic diet. People in the low-carb group ended up burning 300 *more* calories per day than those on a low-fat diet and 200 more calories a day than those on a full-time low-glycemic diet—without exercising any longer or harder.[4] That's like exercising vigorously for an extra hour a week!

Third, the toning/strength-training moves in the 2-Day Diet Workout challenge your muscles to stay strong, allowing you to hold on to more muscle mass and even build more of it as you lose weight.

The result? In contrast with conventional diets, the 2-Day Diet enabled our test panelists to lose more body fat and less muscle. Average weight loss was 9.1 pounds—and 7.5 pounds of that was body fat! Seven panelists built lean muscle as they lost weight, and 13 improved their muscle-to-fat ratio. Good deal!

THE PERFECT PLAN!

The 2-Day Diet is right for you if:

■ You've ever started a diet, only to give up after getting off track and eating the "wrong" foods.

■ You've lost weight only to gain it back at least once in the past.

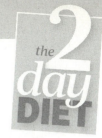

The Beauty of the Buddy System

Sara Phillips and Renee Guzenski, who work together at a nature conservancy in southeastern Pennsylvania, were intrigued when they heard that Rodale—the publisher of this book—was looking for volunteers to try out a new weight-loss concept. They signed on, then buddied up, and the pounds rolled off.

"I couldn't have done it without Sara," says Renee, 40, who lost 13.25 pounds on the 2-Day Diet.

"Same here," says Sara, 64, who lost 16.6 pounds. "We see each other every day and helped each other keep going. It was just more fun this way."

Renee's an accounting associate. Sara's an executive administrative assistant. Their desks are near each other, and their work schedules are in sync—so they can eat lunch and a snack at the same time. These friends turned their 2-Day Diet meals into little adventures. "I brought ingredients for some lunches and snacks, Sara brought ingredients for others," Renee says. "Every Monday we had the Turkey Panini from the 5-Day Jump Start menu. We made them here and heated them up in the office toaster oven."

The pair also decided to split up the daily snack that's always part of this eating plan. "We had half in the morning, half in the afternoon," Sara says. "Our favorite snack was the 2 ounces of Cheddar cheese and half of an apple. At 11 o'clock we'd say, 'Okay, it's time for our snack.' We'd do the same at 3 in the afternoon."

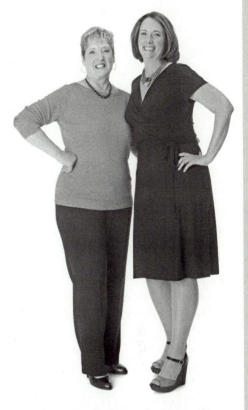

Sara and Renee started other weight-loss traditions, too. They decided to designate Mondays and Tuesdays as their low-carb days each week. And they found an easy solution to the midafternoon desire for a sweet. "We craved something sweet in the afternoon, so we bought diet root beer and diet cream soda," Sara says. "We'd go down and get cups of ice, pour a glass of diet soda, and enjoy it together. It was just enough to take the edge off that craving—and keep us on track."

- You need the flexibility of a plan that makes room for meals out, vacations, days when there's no time to cook, and the needs of a spouse, partner, kids, and other family members.

- You're tired of following restrictive diets for weeks and weeks.

- You just don't have time to exercise every day.

- You want to lower your risk for major health threats such as diabetes, heart disease, stroke, high blood pressure, and more.

What can you expect during the 2-Day Diet? First, remember a few simple numbers: Eat 50 grams of carbohydrates a day on the 2 days a week of your choice. Eat reasonable portions of healthy foods the other days. Add the 2-Day Diet Workout. Follow the plan for 6 weeks. The details:

PHASE 1: THE 5-DAY JUMP START

- Eat three low-carb meals plus one low-carb snack each day.

- Have 50 grams of carbohydrates per day. Carb counts average 15 grams per meal and 5 grams per snack.

- Follow our delicious meal plans and easy recipes for breakfast, lunch, dinner, and snacks. You'll develop a repertoire of low-carb meals and dishes you can prepare in a flash in Phase 2. You can also use the quick low-carb suggestions and dining out strategies in Chapter 9. Just be sure your daily carb total is 50 grams.

PHASE 2: THE 2-DAY DIET

- Eat low-carb 2 days a week. You choose the days that work best for you. Your low-carb days don't have to be consecutive, and you can choose the same, or different, days each week.

TEST PANELIST TIP: *Repeat Your Favorite Breakfast*

Diane Mann made mornings easy with a breakfast "special" that became her go-to meal on busy weekdays. "Every morning I had turkey bacon and eggs and a piece of low-carb toast," she says. "I could make it quickly, and it took the guesswork out of my morning meal. What could be easier?"

■ Enjoy healthy portions of a wide variety of good-for-you foods by following our meal plan and suggestions the other 5 days a week.

■ On low-carb days, aim for a total of 50 grams of carbohydrates or fewer. Spread your carbs—vegetables, low-carb bread, fruit, and dairy products—throughout the day. In general, go for an average of 15 grams of carbs at each meal plus 5 grams of carbs for your daily snack.

And follow the 2-Day Diet Workout, starting with the 5-Day Jump Start. This plan features two kinds of workouts, totaling 45 minutes each:

■ **Day 1: Peak Interval Workout plus Endurance Toning.** Alternate supershort, 15-second bursts of higher-intensity activity with longer, 45-second recovery periods as you walk, ride your exercise bike, swim, or do exercises in your own living room. You'll blast fat and calories, lose pounds, and get energized in just 30 minutes (including 5 minutes to warm up and 5 minutes to cool down at the end). Also do the workout's 15-minute Endurance Toning Routine, using light hand weights as you move through five multimuscle strength-training exercises.

■ **Day 2: Tempo Interval Workout plus Power Toning.** Exercise at a medium-high intensity for 4 minutes at a time, then recover at a lower, easier pace for 1 minute, then repeat. You'll build stamina while losing weight with this 30-minute routine, which includes a 5-minute warmup and a 5-minute cooldown. Add the 15-minute Power Toning Routine, which uses heavier weights as you perform multimuscle strength-training moves.

Ready to start the easiest weight-loss plan ever? Read on to learn more about the plan—then get started today!

Mary Banyas

AGE: 52

HEIGHT: 5'2"

POUNDS LOST: 11.2

INCHES LOST: 20.50—
including 9.25 inches from her waist and 3 inches from her hips

HEALTH UPGRADE: Mary lost 17.4 pounds of body fat and added 6.2 pounds of muscle. Her blood pressure and LDL cholesterol fell to healthier levels. She's got more energy, too.

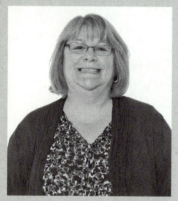

BEFORE

"Come On, Nana! Let's Play Kickball!"

"When you're successful at losing weight, you just feel better about yourself," notes Mary Banyas, an administrative assistant in the marketing department of a large medical center. "I was amazed at how quickly I lost inches and how quickly people started noticing the changes after I started the 2-Day Diet."

The proud grandmother of a 10-year-old grandson and 7-year-old granddaughter, Mary soon found herself up and moving with the kids, too. "I felt more comfortable without all the weight around my waist," she says. "And because I made a commitment to regular exercise, I felt stronger and more energetic."

So instead of sitting and watching her grandchildren play, she found herself joining in—and having a lot of fun. "They wouldn't let me sit down anymore," she says, laughing. "They would say, 'Come on, Nana! Let's play kickball! Let's take a walk!' So we did!" Mary and the kids took hikes in the woods, walked her daughter's dog, Maya, a mixed-breed rescue pooch, and played games on the lawn.

Mary also headed off to her favorite Zumba class regularly. It delivered a mix of higher- and lower-intensity movements that fit the recommendations in the 2-Day Diet Workout. But it was a perfect fit for lots of other reasons, too—including the lively music and dance moves she loves, the convenience (the class is within walking distance of her house, a plus when you're trying to exercise and work full-time), and the fact that her daughter joined her. "We're very close," Mary says. "I love spending time with my family."

For Mary, the flexibility made the 2-Day Diet work. "This wasn't really a diet," she says. "You could adjust it to fit what you needed, and that made all the difference. I've tried low-carb diets in the past, but having to stick with it every single day was so hard. I got headaches and really missed fruit. On this plan, it's easy to eat low-carb just 2 days a week—and it even includes foods like fruit that you don't usually see on a low-carb plan."

Take dining out, something Mary and her husband enjoy. "I discovered that eating out was easy if I ordered meals that were like the meals in the plan," she says. "I might order a Cobb salad without the bacon and take half home, so that I stuck with a healthy portion. If we went to Texas Roadhouse, I'd get sirloin kebabs and a salad. That usually comes with rice and a vegetable, but I'd ask for two veggies—plain, to make sure they weren't cooked in butter."

That's a big contrast to the chicken wings, ribs, and mashed potatoes she often ordered in the past. "Now I might have a tiny bite just to taste the ribs, but that's it," she says. "I love the taste of food. Now I'm enjoying better-quality food that's good for me, and I savor it more. I'm listening to what my body's telling me when I eat—what makes me feel good, what really doesn't."

Losing inches opened up a whole new wardrobe that had been waiting for Mary in the back of her closet. "I went on a cruise about a month before starting the program, and my summer clothes really didn't fit well, but they fit me fine now," she says. "My favorite jeans fit comfortably now, too—after all, I dropped a full size!"

CHAPTER 2

Weight-Loss *power*

2 + 2 = A Slimmer You

On the 2-Day Diet, good things really do come in very small packages. You've already read about these amazing results, but they bear repeating, because they're also our promise to you: Our test panelists dropped an average of 9.1 pounds—including 7.5 pounds of body fat. They trimmed an average of 10.9 inches from their waistlines, hips, thighs, chest, and upper arms combined—including an average of 3.6 inches from their waistlines and 2.3 from their hips. *You* will lose pounds, fat, and inches on this plan, too.

They slid into their skinny jeans, got back into size 10 summer capris that had been languishing at the back of the closet, and started wearing form-fitting tops again—and one panelist needed last-minute tailoring to have a bridesmaid's dress taken in, just in time for a friend's wedding. Test panelist Michelle Sparr told us her dress was a little snug at the start of the diet but was too loose through the torso just a month later! Michelle proudly brought a photo to her final weigh-in— in it, she's wearing the strapless, daffodil yellow dress, smiling happily as she dances with her father at the reception. She looked, and said she felt, beautiful.

The plan responsible for these amazing changes couldn't be shorter or simpler: just 2 days of low-carb eating a week plus two superefficient weekly workouts.

"It was really easy," says Michelle, who lost 3.2 pounds and a whopping 6 inches from her waist. "I've never counted carbs before, and it really opened my eyes to the extra carbs in so many foods. I've found new ways to stay full and satisfied without all the bread and pasta and sweetened yogurt, and the results are terrific."

For Anne Marie York, who lost 6.8 pounds and trimmed 4 inches from her waist and 3.75 inches from her hips, the plan cleared up years of diet confusion so that she could finally lose weight. "For the past couple of years, I felt like I was exercising as much as I possibly could, but something was missing," she says. "I knew how to exercise. I'd gone to plenty of classes and even worked with a personal trainer. But the eating part was missing, and I didn't know what to do. You listen to all these things on TV and read about new diets in magazines—eat this, don't eat that, follow this plan, follow that plan—but you end up just feeling overwhelmed by all the different diet choices. This plan works for me because it's based on foods I eat and like already, it's simple, and it's not even a diet. It's just a healthy way to eat all the time!"

Mary Banyas lost 11.2 pounds and 9.25 inches from her waist. As a result, she's wearing a smaller pants size. "That's awesome," she says. "Eleven pounds is a lot of weight to lose in just 6 weeks. Think about picking up a 10-pound bag of potatoes—it's heavy! And I lost a pound more than that!"

Renee Guzenski had eight pairs of dress pants that stopped fitting her when she gained weight. After losing 13.25 pounds in 6 weeks on the 2-Day Diet, she's wearing them again. "And jeans that were skintight at the start of the program are now loose on me," she says. Her co-worker Sara Phillips, who followed the program with her, lost 16.6 pounds and can once again wear pants, suits, summer capris, and a favorite black dress, all of which had become way too snug. "My belts for my pants went from being pretty tight on the first notch to being down to the third notch and still loose," she says. "And that black dress is so nice. It used

TEST PANELIST TIP: *Crunch Time*

Nancy Barnes missed bread and crackers at first, then found that wrapping sandwich fillings in lettuce leaves and dipping celery or cucumber slices into salsa and other dips was uniquely satisfying. "I found that I really love foods that crunch," she says. "I always thought you had to have crackers with your cheese, but it turns out that anything crunchy—like cucumbers or celery—is just as good. I also liked almonds mixed into my yogurt, for the same reason. You really feel like you're eating something substantial."

to look like my belly and my butt stuck out too much in it, but now it looks great!" (We agree—Phillips brought the dress to her final weigh-in and looked fabulous in it.)

Sharon Spitz lost 7.8 pounds of body fat and trimmed 7 all-over inches thanks to careful eating and a new commitment to exercise—including the 2-Day Diet interval-training and toning workouts. "I put on more lean muscle as I lost body fat, so the number on the scale didn't change," she says. "But weight is just a number. The body fat and the inches are truly the important picture. They determine how you look and even how you feel."

In just 6 weeks, you can achieve similar results on the 2-Day Diet. It's easy to follow—and every bit of this super-easy, no-slipups plan is designed to keep you on track and losing pounds with a minimum of effort. It's the easiest diet ever. Behind it are research-proven principles that ramp up healthy weight loss while minimizing the factors that make so many other diets fail.

INSIDE THE 2-DAY DIET EATING PLAN

The plan couldn't be simpler.

- **2 days a week, enjoy healthy, tasty, low-carbohydrate meals plus a snack.** Meals focus on lean protein, good fats, nonstarchy vegetables, and enough whole grains, dairy, and even fruit in the mix for satisfaction and optimal nutrition. You can pick any days of the week to go low-carb, and the days don't have to be consecutive. Overall, you'll eat 50 grams of carbohydrates a day—about 15 grams per meal, plus 5 grams in a healthy snack.

- **5 days a week, enjoy regular-carb eating.** Lean protein and good fats are still key players, but now you'll enjoy more grains, fruits, a wider variety of vegetables (like corn, potatoes, and legumes such as red, white, and navy beans), and even dessert.

> **TEST PANELIST TIP:** *Naturally Sweet*
>
> Michelle Sparr loves yogurt for breakfast but was shocked by the carb count in her favorite fruit flavors. "I switched to plain Greek yogurt and added fruit, but it really wasn't sweet enough," she says. "I decided to try organic stevia, a low-calorie, low-carb sweetener. I sprinkle a little in my yogurt. It makes it tastier without any aftertaste. That—plus the sweetness of raspberries or strawberries or blueberries I toss in—is delicious and filling."

Weight-loss magic? It seems like a dream come true. You get the benefits of a full-time diet in less than half the time—and without the downsides that end too many weight-loss attempts early or lead to regain. The following are some things you won't do on the 2-Day Diet:

- No slogging through weeks and months of deprivation. Diet just 2 days a week, eat normally the other 5!

- No need to struggle back after a slipup. This plan is slip-proof!

- No worries about fitting a diet and exercise plan into a date book already packed with family commitments, work, meals away from home, parties, holidays, vacations, and—let's be honest—days when you just want to take a break. You choose your 2 diet days!

- No more "post-diet slump"—the critical time just after a formal diet ends, when loosening the reins sets the stage for regain, remorse, and more regain. You can add back 1 or 2 low-carb days a week to quickly lose pounds if they creep back on. And continuing to follow the plan's satisfying, regular-carb healthy meals assures a lifetime at a healthy weight!

The 2-Day Diet eating plan melts fat thanks to a revolutionary, proven mix of low-carb days plus "regular" days. (For best results, add the 2-Day Diet Workout to torch more calories and fat while building sleek, metabolism-boosting muscle.) This eating plan is powered by decades of scientific research in the amazing fields of part-time dieting and low-carb dieting. By combining these two weight-loss strategies, you get the best of both, without the downsides that derail other diets. Here's the story of the two weight-loss philosophies that meet in this revolutionary plan.

PART-TIME DIETS—CIGARS, COFFEE . . . AND DESPERATION AT THE START

No 21st-century doctor would recommend a diet of black coffee and cigars. But in the early 1960s, American physicians looking for a new way to help obese patients lose weight experimented with a part-time diet strategy called "intermittent fasting." It's not something we'd recommend. Extremely overweight women and men checked into the hospital for medically supervised fasts lasting from 1 to 15 days. Afterward, they continued fasting for 1 or 2 days a week at home, sipping water, tea, coffee—and in one case study documented in the journal *Transactions of the American Clinical and Climatological Association* in 1962, an inveterate smoker was allowed to puff cigars with his cups of black coffee.[1]

Volunteers in one study, and presumably their doctors, were desperate to find a solution to stubborn and dangerous obesity. "Most of these patients had abandoned hope that they could reduce on diets that would reduce normal individuals," a study researcher from Pennsylvania Hospital in Philadelphia wrote at the time. They hadn't slimmed down on low-calorie diets. Weight-loss drugs of the 1950s and 1960s, exercise, visits to psychiatrists, and "bizarre diets" had failed them, too. So part-time dieting offered new hope. Of 109 volunteers in that study, just 2 dropped out. Intermittent fasting wasn't easy, but those who stuck with it lost up to 82 pounds. When researchers checked in with them up to $2\frac{1}{2}$ years later, 43 percent had kept the weight off and 17 percent had lost even more.

Well before the obesity epidemic hit America late in the 20th century, this type of extreme on-again, off-again dieting was seen as a solution for a few extremely overweight people. It began turning up in medical journals around the world more and more often in the 1960s and 1970s. In lab studies, it offered big health benefits—mice and rats ended up with healthier hearts[2] and sharper brains.[3] But in humans, there were real drawbacks. It worked for a dedicated few, but over time many people regained their weight and then some. Eastern European researchers noticed that muscles were shrinking in women who fasted and then ate low-calorie meals in repeating 5-day cycles.[4] Fasting for days on end, followed by a break before fasting again, was too difficult for most people. Some researchers even called it "the hunger diet"[5] or "the starvation diet."[6] One risk: Besides having absolutely no taste appeal and being very difficult to stick with, slashing calories this dramatically can shift your metabolism into low-gear "starvation mode," so that you burn fewer calories round the clock. As a result, normal eating could lead to even more weight gain.

Still, the idea of part-time dieting had been launched, although it wasn't ready for prime time.

The Evolution of a Great Idea

As the obesity epidemic took off in the 1990s and first decade of the 21st century, researchers took a second look at part-time diets. They tweaked, tested, and measured the results; tweaked a little more; discovered a bunch of intriguing benefits; and finally struck gold. Here's how the concept of "on and off" dieting advanced—and the exciting discoveries that inspired the plan in this book:

Discovery #1: Part-time diets keep your metabolism revved and don't lead to

overeating. One of the biggest questions was, Won't I just overeat on "regular" days and lose all the benefits? Another concern was, Do part-time diets lower metabolism the way a full-time, reduced-calorie diet can? The answer to both questions, it turns out, is no.

In one 2005 study from the Pennington Biomedical Research Center in Baton Rouge, Louisiana, researchers wanted to know whether fasting every other day would lead to overeating on "off days." If it did, then all that work and hunger would be a waste. So they put 16 women and men on an alternate-day fast for 22 days—11 days of no food, interspersed with days when they could eat whatever they wanted in any quantity. They were even told to take second helpings on off days so they wouldn't lose weight, essentially giving them permission to pig out. The surprising result: Despite eating extra on those off days, volunteers lost an average of 3 to 4 pounds.

This study turned up two body chemistry bonuses for part-time dieting. Study volunteers' resting metabolic rate—the number of calories their bodies burned round the clock—didn't lower as it can with more extreme diets. And an important longevity gene called SIRT1, which protects cells from the damaging effects of stress, was more active by the end of the study.[7] But there was a big downside: Participants felt hungry and irritable all the time on fast days.[8] Reluctantly, the scientists concluded that skipping meals every other day might not become a popular solution for the nation's weight problem.

Discovery #2: Part-time diets reduce insulin levels and insulin resistance. One side effect of weight gain (especially belly fat), lack of exercise, and a high-fat diet is insulin resistance. Your body has trouble absorbing blood sugar. This raises your risk for diabetes, heart disease, cancer, and other health conditions—and

---

TEST PANELIST TIP: *Inspire Yourself with Music*

As the mother of two preschoolers, Sharon Spitz hears lots of Muppets music at home, and she's added some of their songs to her iPod playlist. "I listened a lot to the song 'Just One Person' by the Muppeteers," she says. "It's all about believing in yourself. It was perfect for this workout—it taught me to believe in myself. My legs were sore sometimes after the elliptical trainer, but I got stronger and had more stamina."

Spitz also listened to podcasts of radio programs that she doesn't always have time for at home. "One of my favorites is *Wait Wait . . . Don't Tell Me!*" she says. "It keeps me laughing and makes the time go faster."

can make weight loss more difficult, especially at midlife. It also means your body pumps out more and more insulin to force blood sugar (glucose) into cells, and the extra insulin may interfere with fat burning.

In Denmark, researchers wondered whether a new kind of eating could help reverse insulin resistance. Their big question: We humans evolved to survive, and even thrive, in a tough, prehistoric world of feast and famine. Would re-creating those conditions make 21st-century humans a little healthier? To find out, eight normal-weight guys fasted on and off for 14 days in a 2005 study from the University of Copenhagen. The result: Their bodies processed blood sugar better than before—a body chemistry bonus that could help overweight people lose weight.[9]

Discovery #3: You don't have to starve on "diet days." Nobody wants a diet that promises you'll feel hungry, light-headed, and cranky half the time. Was there a better way? To find out, Louisiana State University researchers tested a part-time diet that (finally!) let dieters eat every day but cut calories dramatically every *other* day. Would "alternate-day calorie restriction" lead to weight loss? Could people stick with it? And would it free them from the need to count calories (they noted that figuring out portion sizes and calorie counts isn't easy)? Ten overweight people embarked on an 8-week diet that featured a skinny 320 to 380 calories every other day. They ate what they wanted on off days.

The result: Study volunteers lost 8 percent of their body weight, about 18.5 pounds. Their moods improved. Hunger scores ranged between 5 and 6 on a scale of 1 to 10 on low-calorie days throughout the study—just slightly higher than on the days when they were able to eat what they wanted. The body chemistry bonus: Their bodies "listened" better to the satisfaction hormone leptin.[10] Alternate-day calorie restriction "does not result in a sustained overactivation of the hunger response," the scientists said. (Volunteers in this study all had asthma; the diet also improved their breathing, perhaps by reducing inflammation.)

Discovery #4: You can eat real food on diet days. Whew. Things looked up for part-time dieters when researchers from the University of Illinois at Chicago

---

TEST PANELIST TIP: *Turn Low-Carb Noodles into a Feast*

Dale Honig found a great way to turn shirataki noodles into a delicious meal. "I doctored them up," she says. "After cooking the noodles according to the package directions, I'd sauté some greens such as Swiss chard, plus a little garlic, fresh tomato, and Bermuda onion in olive oil. I'd pour that over the noodles, then add a bit of skim milk and Parmesan cheese to create a little sauce. It's delicious!"

tested an alternate-day plan that let study volunteers eat a "real meal" on diet days and stick with a reasonable eating plan on off days. It still wasn't a breeze. Dieters were limited to one meal—a hearty lunch, with dishes like chicken fettuccine, enchiladas, or pizza—no breakfast or dinner on their diet days. Still, they lost an average of 12 pounds in 10 weeks.[11]

THE 2-DAY DIET BREAKTHROUGH

Part-time dieting had come a long way, marching from starvation (no thanks!) to real meals, but it was still a mighty tough plan to stick with. Could you live on meal replacement shakes or just one meal a day at lunchtime, every other day, for weeks on end? We couldn't. Even the University of Illinois researchers who devised the "real meal" diet wondered if their volunteers could have done it without regular, motivational check-ins with a dietitian. Was there an even better way? Scientists in the United Kingdom suspected the answer was yes and began looking into the "express" version of the part-time diet: 2-day dieting.

Their first question: How would a 2-day diet stack up against a full-time diet? For 6 months, 107 overweight and obese British women followed one of two diets. Half ate about 1,500 calories per day, 7 days a week, of healthy foods (plenty of produce, lean protein, good fats, a smattering of whole grains, and low-fat dairy products). The other half followed an extremely low-calorie diet 2 days a week and ate what they liked the rest of the time. The meal plan for low-calorie days was 2 pints of low-fat milk, 4 servings of vegetables, one small piece of fruit, a salty low-calorie drink, and a multivitamin.

The results were surprising. After 6 months, the low-calorie group lost 14.5 pounds, while the full-time dieters dropped 12 pounds. Both groups also saw cholesterol and blood pressure levels improve. Interestingly, the low-calorie group saw bigger blood sugar benefits: Their bodies became less insulin resistant, so cells absorbed blood sugar more readily.[12] The women, many of whom were at high risk for breast cancer, also saw levels of hormones related to breast cancer risk fall. "The findings are important because they could give people who are overweight an alternative way to lose weight," the researchers said.

The only catch? The milk-and-produce diet menu plan wasn't exactly yummy. So the researchers went back to the lab in search of a tastier alternative. Their aha moment: low-carb diet days instead of severely calorie-restricted diet days. Low-carbohydrate diets—which limit foods containing added and natural sugars and starches (such as sweets, bread, noodles, and even fruit, dairy, and vegetables)—were already proven to subtract pounds and improve the way the body processes blood sugar. Would 2 low-carb days per week get results?

They put 115 overweight women on one of three diets: a conventional, reduced-calorie plan (1,500 calories) 7 days a week; a low-carbohydrate plan (600 calories) 2 days a week; or a low-carbohydrate plan that focused on lean protein and healthy fats but didn't count calories 2 days a week. Volunteers followed the plans for 3 months, then moved into a maintenance phase: The full-time dieters increased their calories to 1,900 a day. The part-time dieters followed their low-carb plans 1 day a week; on other days, they ate a reasonable, healthy diet.

The outcome wowed the weight-loss world. The low-carb, part-time dieters lost more weight—an average of 11 to 12 pounds versus 8 pounds for full-time dieters. More of their shed weight was body fat, too—an average of 9 pounds compared with 5.5 for full-time dieters. That's a double benefit, because losing body fat improves health, and holding on to more muscle during weight loss keeps your metabolism revved for better weight maintenance. There's also evidence that the low-carb dieters lost more belly fat: Their waistlines shrank 2 inches versus 1.4 inches for full-time dieters. Part-time dieters also had better insulin sensitivity, a sign of reduced risk for breast cancer and other major health conditions.[13]

The verdict? "Restricting carbohydrates 2 days per week may be a better dietary approach than a standard, daily calorie-restricted diet for weight loss and prevention of breast cancer and other diseases," the researchers said.

We said *wow*. The results inspired us to create the plan in this book.

LOW-CARB, 2 DAYS: THE BEST OF BOTH WORLDS

Low-carb diets have been on bookstore shelves and in the news for more than a decade now. Everyone's read or seen stories on TV or knows someone who claims to have lost big by loading his or her plate with protein and fat while steering clear of refined carbohydrates in sweets, sodas, and white bread and even cutting back on whole grains, fruit, and starchy veggies. In recent years, "eco-carb diets" have replaced old-fashioned steak, cheese, and butter meal plans with healthier lean proteins like chicken and fish and good fats found in nuts, olive and canola oils, and avocado.

Normally, your body's preferred source of fuel is blood sugar (glucose) from the carbohydrates you eat. Whole grain bread, chocolate cake, your breakfast banana and oatmeal, and veggies (from starchy types such as corn and lima beans to tomatoes, spinach, and carrots) all contain carbohydrates, as do dairy products. Your body breaks them all down and converts them into glucose, which is absorbed into your bloodstream. The hormone insulin tells cells throughout your body to absorb glucose into the cell, where it's burned for energy every time you go out for a walk, pick up a child, hit the dance floor, or simply take a breath.

What happens when you cut back on carbs? Insulin levels drop, opening the door for your body to burn more fat for energy. Although this claim is still regarded as controversial, in recent research studies low-carb diets really have torched more body fat and belly fat (the kind that boosts risk for diabetes, heart disease, and some cancers) than low-fat diets with the same number of calories.

- In one study from Johns Hopkins University, presented at an American Heart Association conference in 2012, low-carb dieters lost more total fat, more abdominal fat, and more weight than people who followed a low-fat diet with the same number of daily calories.[14]

- Low-carb diets bested other types of diets for maintaining weight loss in a new Children's Hospital Boston study of 21 overweight and obese young women and men who'd just completed a weight-loss program. Low-carb eating helped them keep the weight off because it kept their metabolism revved higher. Study volunteers on a low-carb eating plan burned an average of 300 *more* calories per day than those on low-fat diets (and 150 more calories per day than those on a low-glycemic diet)—without having to exercise any longer or harder.[15] The diet seems to help by maintaining muscle mass and encouraging cells to burn more of the body's biggest fuel sources: fatty acids and blood sugar.

- People on low-carb diets burned more of the fat stored in their liver than those on a low-calorie diet in a 2009 study from the University of Texas Southwestern Advanced Imaging Research Center. A fatty liver is a surprisingly common yet often overlooked "side effect" of being overweight that affects up to one-third of American adults. They also burned more overall body fat.[16]

- And in a 2011 study from the University of Alabama at Birmingham involving 69 overweight women and men, those on a low-carb diet lost 11 percent more

TEST PANELIST TIP: *Leftovers into Lunch*

"My husband wasn't on the diet with me, so I'd cut the recipes in half," says Mary Banyas. "I'd have half for dinner, put the rest in a container, and save it for lunch the next day. I loved getting two meals out of one night of cooking. I'd do the same if we ate out—so easy."

deep abdominal fat and 4 percent more overall body fat than those on a high-carbohydrate, low-fat diet with the same number of calories.[17]

Advantage: 5 "Off Days" Every Week!

Getting your low-carb eating out of the way in 2 days each week means you've got 5 days for more liberal eating—days when pasta, sandwiches, potatoes, and even dessert and pancakes are on the menu. Breaks get you past any sense of deprivation. They work around one of the downsides of full-time low-carb eating, especially for women: low energy and low moods.

Several test panelists told us they'd tried full-time low-carb diets in the past but found they were tough to stick with. "Eating low-carb and lots of protein every single day is difficult," says test panelist Sara Phillips. "Two days a week is so much easier."

Breaks are a proven secret weapon for weight loss, as University of Pittsburgh researchers discovered when they tried to study diet relapses. In a 2003 experiment with 142 overweight women and men, one-third dieted continuously for 11 long months while the others were told to go on diet vacations.[18] No counting calories or stepping on the bathroom scale. One group took a 6-week break, the other took three 2-week breaks. After 11 months, all three groups had lost strikingly similar amounts of weight. The researchers suspected that continuous diets led to more cheating, while those who got a break were able to follow their plans to the letter when they resumed. Breaks don't ruin a diet—they can help you stick with it!

Advantage: Less Hunger, More Satisfaction

From steak with blue cheese dressing to walnut-crusted chicken breasts, the high-satisfaction proteins and good fats you'll enjoy on low-carb days stave off hunger and boost satisfaction. You even get fruit, whole grains, and dairy products—foods that are usually limited or even off-limits on full-time low-carb diets. You also get a snack every day. Low-carb eating keeps your appetite in check and your tummy from growling for three reasons.

First, proteins such as chicken, lean beef and pork, fish, eggs, and tofu take longer to digest than many carbohydrates. Same goes for the good fats you'll enjoy, including nuts, nut butters, avocado, and olive and canola oils.

Second, low-carb diets are proven to suppress hunger pangs.[19] Steadier blood sugar after meals and lower insulin levels are part of the reason, report University of Alabama at Birmingham researchers. They made the discovery by testing the blood of 30 people who followed low- and high-carb diets for 4 weeks. The low-carbers felt fuller after a test meal—and stayed full longer.[20]

Third, 2-day dieting makes your whole body more sensitive to leptin, the satisfaction hormone. Many people battling excess pounds are leptin resistant—their bodies make plenty of this nifty chemical, but their cells no longer pay attention to it. While leptin resistance won't make you fat, once you're overweight it can become a formidable obstacle to losing weight. A high-fat diet, too little exercise, too much stress, and too little sleep contribute to leptin resistance, too.[21]

Researchers who've studied 2-day diets have found that leptin levels drop on the diet. That's a good thing, because it means your body needs less leptin in order to turn appetite off.

Advantage: You Burn More Fat, Less Muscle

One of the biggest problems with weight-loss diets is that they don't discriminate between puffy, bulky, unhealthy fat and lean, toned, calorie-gobbling muscle—both come off as you lose weight. But losing muscle can slow your resting metabolic rate, the number of calories your body burns round the clock. A slowed-down metabolism is one reason people hit diet plateaus; it also makes weight maintenance more difficult. As your metabolism slows, your body burns fewer calories throughout the day, which means you'd have to eat even less food than you might expect to maintain a new, lower weight. *Not* easy.

A 2-day low-carb diet, though, minimizes muscle loss while maximizing fat loss. In the British study we described earlier in this chapter, people who ate this way lost 11 to 12 pounds—and 9 to 9.5 pounds of it were fat. Following a full-time calorie-controlled diet led to an 8-pound weight loss, with just 5.5 pounds from

(continued on page 30)

Nancy Barnes

AGE: 65

HEIGHT: 5'4"

POUNDS LOST: 8.4

INCHES LOST: 9.25— including 2.25 inches from her hips

HEALTH UPGRADE: Nancy's BMI fell from 28.9 to a healthier 27.5. Her LDL cholesterol dropped 35 points, her "good" HDL cholesterol rose 7 points, and her already healthy blood pressure fell to an even healthier level.

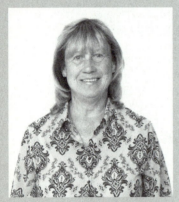

BEFORE

"I Really Feel the Energy Difference"

Nancy Barnes, a retired massage therapist, doesn't have a bathroom scale. So when her clothes started fitting her better several weeks into the program, she knew it was working. "I don't want to be obsessed with the number on the scale," she explains. "Other things are more important—like whether or not I'm eating well, exercising regularly, and staying healthy. I know myself pretty well. If my clothes are looser, I'm losing weight and inches."

The surprise for Nancy was just how much 6 weeks on the 2-Day Diet improved two important measures of heart health: her cholesterol and her blood pressure levels. "I haven't been able to get my cholesterol down below 300 in a while," she says. "There's a lot of heart disease and stroke in my family. So I loved discovering that I can still bring my numbers down with diet and exercise, which I have not been able to do in the past. That's really significant for me."

Another discovery: Nancy found she didn't miss higher-carbohydrate foods like bread, chips, and crackers if she substituted vegetable edibles on her low-carb days. Lettuce leaves replaced bread for sandwiches; cool cucumber slices stood in for crackers. She also found she could reproduce the "comfort food" qualities of starchy foods like mashed potatoes and noodles with veggies such as zucchini and cauliflower.

"The plan made me aware of the need to check food labels for carbs," she says. "I didn't realize that higher-carb foods, especially refined carbs and added sugars, can lead to sugar highs and lows that leave you with low energy and more cravings. This plan has permanently changed the way I eat." One new habit: Instead of sugary, high-carb granola for breakfast, she'll have plain nonfat yogurt dressed up with fruit, nuts, and perhaps a sprinkle of the natural, no-calorie sweetener stevia.

Nancy adapted the 2-Day Diet meal plans to help control her cholesterol level by choosing egg whites or an egg substitute instead of whole eggs and by opting for low-fat cheese. "I did have a little bit of butter, which was nice to see on the plan because it tastes so good," she says. "And I still enjoyed cheese and milk, but I made sure to choose low-fat varieties."

And as she made all those good choices, she tracked them with a food log. "I was pretty religious about it," she says. "I noted my carbs, and I wrote down everything I ate. That really made me conscious of what I put in my body."

The result? More energy—and plenty of compliments. "I really felt the energy difference thanks to eating fewer carbs," she says. "I slept better, and people who didn't even know I was on a diet have said I look like I've lost weight and that I look great. That makes me feel really good."

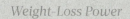

fat. Other studies of part-time diets have had similar findings.[22] The result: You're slimmer and maintain a higher metabolic rate. Your body burns more calories round the clock. (Adding the strength-building moves in our 2-Day Diet Workout will help you hold on to more muscle and even build up more sleek, toned muscle.)

This is especially good news for anyone who's already celebrated a 30th, 40th, or 50th birthday (or beyond!). We all naturally lose about 1 percent of our muscle mass a year in middle age. Between 40 and 50, that could mean the loss of 10 percent of muscle mass—and a 3 to 6 percent drop in metabolism.[23] In contrast, hanging on to as much muscle as possible during weight loss—and adding more through 2 days a week of weight training, as you will on the 2-Day Diet plan—could increase your metabolism by 7 to 8 percent. You'll look better, feel more energetic, and have an easier time losing pounds and keeping them off.[24]

And as our test panelists quickly discovered, this brilliant eating strategy is also an all-round health booster. Discover how it can benefit your heart, your blood sugar, and more in Chapter 3.

CHAPTER 3

Health power

The winning formula behind the 2-Day Diet—2 low-carb days plus 5 regular-carb days each week—will help you slide into your skinniest jeans with room to spare. But the benefits don't stop there. This plan's unique nutrient balance delivers impressive bodywide health advantages, too.

Our test panelists were wowed by the results: Cholesterol, triglycerides, blood pressure, and blood sugar levels dropped. Belly fat—a potent risk factor for diabetes, heart disease, cancer, and even dementia and brittle bones—melted. *Every test panelist* got at least two of the following health bonuses as measured by "before" and "after" blood tests, blood pressure readings, and tape measure checks:

■ **Lower LDL cholesterol.** Twelve panelists saw levels of this heart-threatening blood fat fall—by as much as 35 points. This is the fat that clogs artery walls, leading to heart attacks and strokes, so less is definitely better. Nancy Barnes's LDLs fell from 225 to 190 mg/dL; Kim Rosario's LDLs dropped 7 points, while her husband, Luis Rosario, saw his drop by 23 points! That really helps your heart and arteries, because every 1 percent drop in LDL cholesterol (equal to 1.5 mg/dL if your LDLs are now 150 mg/dL) lowers your risk for heart disease by 1 percent.[1]

■ **Better blood pressure.** Eleven panelists saw drops in their blood pressure by the end of the program. Five even moved from borderline high numbers back to a healthier range. Kathy Rocchetti's blood pressure fell from a borderline high 138/80 to a healthy 120/78, and Mary Banyas saw her numbers drop from a borderline high 130/88 to a healthier 112/84. Avoiding high blood pressure is crucial; this common problem (90 percent of us are at risk after age 55!) raises heart disease risk 75 percent and triggers half of all strokes.

- **Healthier blood sugar.** Eight panelists saw their fasting blood glucose levels fall—an indication that their bodies were processing fuel (blood sugar) from the food they ate in a healthier way. Anne Morris's blood sugar fell from a troubling 111 to 99; Dale Honig's dropped from 95 to 88. Lower blood sugar levels can indicate that your body is more sensitive to insulin, the hormone that commands cells to absorb blood sugar. That's a good thing. Today, many of us are insulin resistant, which lowers our ability to use food efficiently and boosts our risk for diabetes, heart disease, dementia, and even some types of cancer.

- **Trimmer triglycerides.** Ten panelists saw levels of this blood fat fall—by as much as 155 points. At high levels (over 150 mg/dL), this blood fat raises risk for heart attacks and strokes. Cutting back on refined carbohydrates is an expert-endorsed way to rein in triglycerides, so it's no surprise that this low-carb eating plan helped. Some big winners: Anne Morris, whose triglycerides fell from a high of 282 to a healthy 127; and Matt Opatovsky, whose triglycerides dropped from 181 to 144.

- **Banished belly fat.** Meanwhile, the tape measure uncovered another important benefit for our test panel: less of the headline-grabbing menace that's emerging as the *real* link between extra pounds and a wide variety of health problems. That menace is belly fat. You've already read about these amazing improvements in Chapter 1—*each and every test panelist trimmed inches from her or his midsection.* Among the biggest "losers": Mary Banyas slimmed her middle by 9.25 inches; Dale Honig lost 9 inches; Sara Phillips trimmed 5 inches from her waistline; Anne Marie York whittled hers by 4 inches; and her sister, Kathy Rocchetti, trimmed her waist by 4.25 inches.

TEST PANELISTS LOVE THE HEALTH UPGRADES

We all know that there are plenty of health risks we *can't* control. Your age, your gender, the genes you inherited from your parents, your ethnicity, and your past medical history all have a hand in determining your future health. But they're not the last word. Experts estimate, for example, that more than 80 percent of heart disease risk,[2] more than 50 percent of cancer risk,[3] and up to 90 percent of diabetes risk[4] is under your control—and can even be prevented with healthy lifestyle steps. It's great knowing that this easy, delicious plan puts powerful tools for prevention in your hands (and on your plate)!

"The improvements in my blood pressure and blood fats—cholesterol and triglycerides—mean more to me than basically anything else," says Anne Marie York, whose blood pressure fell from 124/80 to a lower, healthier 114/76. Her total cholesterol fell from 211 to 172 (keeping total cholesterol under 200 is a smart health goal), her "bad" LDLs dropped from 131 to 106, and her triglycerides fell from 142 to an even healthier 102. "It was just amazing. I know that not everyone can control their cholesterol with diet alone. Genetics plays a role for many people. But to find out that I can is very empowering."

Real-World Results:
Test Panel Health Improvements

The 18 test panelists who followed the 2-Day Diet for 6 weeks saw a wide range of health improvements, as measured by "before" and "after" blood checks and tape measure checks. Here's how they fared as a group on five key health indicators and why these factors are so important for your health.

Health Indicator	Test Panelists Who Saw an Improvement	Why It Matters
Waist size	100%	A smaller waist means less of the deep abdominal fat that raises your risk for diabetes, heart disease, cancer, dementia, and brittle bones.
Fasting blood sugar	44%	Lower blood sugar levels can be a sign that your body is processing blood sugar more efficiently, cutting your risk for diabetes, heart disease, cancer, and more.
Blood pressure	66%	Healthier blood pressure levels lower your risk for stroke, heart attack, hardening of the arteries, kidney problems, and circulation problems such as peripheral artery disease (constricted circulation in your legs that causes pain and fatigue).
LDL cholesterol	70%	Bringing heart-threatening LDL cholesterol down to a healthier level helps protect against heart attacks and strokes.
Triglycerides	65%	Keeping these blood fats within a healthy range lowers risk for heart attacks and strokes, too.

Her sister, Kathy Rocchetti, was thrilled by the improvement in her own blood pressure numbers. "Health is big for us," she says. "There's a history of heart disease, strokes, and high blood pressure in our family. It's great knowing that exercise and changing your diet can be so beneficial."

Sharon Spitz, a registered nurse, was also happy to see that her LDL cholesterol fell 29 points and her triglycerides dropped 11 points. "The important results go beyond the numbers on the scale," she says. "I lost body fat, ate healthier, and exercised more. It's great to see that these changes can make a healthy difference."

Shannon Miller, who has type 1 diabetes, discovered that blood sugar control was easier on the 2-Day Diet. "I've always been very aware of the carbs that I eat," she explains. "When you have type 1 diabetes, you have to match the carbs you eat with your insulin dose. I needed less insulin on the diet. That's great!"

As a matter of fact, our test panelists enjoyed the slimmer, trimmer look that comes with cosmetic liposuction—plus the amazing health benefits that people who undergo liposuction *don't* experience. (Studies show that, while liposuction can whittle inches from bellies and thighs, it has no impact at all on our overall health.[5]

IT'S ALL ABOUT BALANCE

The 2-Day Diet delivers a built-in health boost because it incorporates two proven healthy-eating strategies in a unique, balanced plan.

- Low-carb eating for a metabolic advantage.
- Low-glycemic eating for more of the nutrients your body needs most.

Here's what science says about the power of each of these approaches—and what the latest research and our test panel results show about the benefits of combining the two.

Metabolic Advantage

Plenty of research shows that low-carbohydrate diets reset your body chemistry in beneficial ways that low-fat and even low-glycemic diets can't. The big news is that eating low-carb just 2 days a week delivers these benefits:

Low-carb beats weight-loss drugs for improving blood pressure. In a recent Duke University study, published in the *Archives of Internal Medicine*, 146 overweight people followed a low-carb diet or took the weight-loss drug orlistat while following a conventional low-calorie diet. Both groups lost weight, but only the low-carb group saw a healthy drop in blood pressure. Half of those on blood pressure drugs were able to cut their doses or stop their medications altogether. "If people have high blood pressure and a weight problem, a low-carbohydrate diet might be a better option than a weight loss medication," the study's lead researcher noted.[6] *The 2-Day Diet advantage:* In our test panel, blood pressure levels fell significantly with 2 days of low-carb dieting.

Healthy low-carb eating beats low-fat diets for improving cholesterol numbers. In the past, low-fat, higher-carbohydrate diets have been touted as the best way to rein in high cholesterol levels. But a growing stack of research suggests that a low-carb diet packed with lean protein and good fats—the type you'll enjoy on the 2-Day Diet—is a better way to go. In one Israeli study, published in the *New England Journal of Medicine*, low-carb diets were better at lowering total cholesterol levels.[7] True, old-fashioned low-carb diets that load up on fat-marbled steaks and greasy cheeseburgers can raise your cholesterol levels and heart disease risk, research shows.[8, 9] But a low-carb plan based on good fats and lean protein (closer to the 2-Day Diet) dropped LDL cholesterol by an average of 13 percent in one recent Canadian study, a reduction that cut risk of heart attack and stroke by 11 percent on average.[10] *The 2-Day Diet advantage:* Our test panelists proved it—2 days of low-carb dieting slashed LDL cholesterol.

Low-carb eating improves blood sugar levels. At the VA Medical Center in Minneapolis, Minnesota, two groups of men with type 2 diabetes followed a diet plan for 5 weeks each. The first group followed a low-carb diet, while the second group maintained a regular diet. At the end of the 5 weeks, the low-carb group had fasting blood sugar 72 points lower than the conventional group, and their A1c levels, a measure of long-term blood sugar control, fell from a too-high 9.8 percent to a slightly high 7.6 percent. Researchers called the low-carb plan "empowering." *The 2-Day Diet advantage:* Test panelists saw improvements in the way their body processed blood sugar, as did volunteers in a British study of a 2-day low-carb diet.[11]

Nutritional Bonus

In Chapter 2, you read about a recent Children's Hospital Boston study that compared low-carb, low-fat, and low-glycemic diets for maintaining weight loss in 21 overweight and obese young women and men. Low-carb was the clear winner, keeping metabolism revved higher so that dieters burned on average 300 more calories per day than those on low-fat diets—without having to exercise any longer or harder.[12] Low-glycemic eating, similar to the 2-Day Diet's "simply healthy" days, came in second, with 150 more calories burned per day than low-fat eating. But you may have heard on the news that the low-carb plan also stressed dieters' bodies, raising markers for heart disease.

That points up an important advantage of the 2-Day Diet: With 2 days of low-carb eating *plus* 5 days of low-glycemic eating per week, this plan gives you the health and weight-loss benefits of *both* eating styles without the downsides of full-time low-carb eating. These downsides include higher levels of inflammatory compounds—which raise risks for diabetes, heart disease, and other health concerns—and lower intake of nutrient-packed whole grains, fruit, dried beans, and higher-carb vegetables such as sweet potatoes, winter squash, and peas as well as root veggies like beets, turnips, and parsnips.

Compare the two approaches. In the Children's Hospital Boston study, the full-time low-carb dieters saw markers of inflammation rise somewhat. Body-wide inflammation boosts heart disease risk and raises odds for diabetes and cancer, too. But in a 2011 study, markers of inflammation *fell* when people ate low-carb just part of the time—2 days a week, as you will on the 2-Day Diet. Why? This discovery is so new that researchers are still looking into it. One likely explanation is that eating low-carb part-time simply doesn't boost levels of inflammatory chemicals in your bloodstream as much as full-time low-carb eating seems to. At the same time, eating more inflammation-cooling foods on regular-carb days—like more servings of fruit, a wider range of vegetables, and more whole grains—goes to work in your body to cool off bodywide chronic inflammation. Plenty of research shows that eating more of these foods lowers levels of harmful, inflammation-boosting compounds.

You'll find some of these foods on your plate at every meal every day during the 2-Day Diet because we know how important they are. On low-carb days, we've made room for fruit and whole grains in addition to plenty of vegetables. Then on regular-carb days, you'll find even more of them. Here's how they help your health:

Loads of fruit and vegetables. Unlike full-time low-carb plans that restrict fruit and even many vegetables, you'll enjoy 7 to 10 daily servings of produce on "simply healthy" days and 4 to 6 servings of specially selected low-carb fruits and vegetables on low-carb days. Fruits and vegetables cool inflammation—in one Harvard School of Public Health study of 486 women published in the *American Journal of Clinical Nutrition*, those who munched the most produce had the lowest levels of an inflammation marker called C-reactive protein.[13] Produce also lowers cancer risk. Broccoli and cauliflower, green leafy vegetables, berries, beans, and winter squash help guard your DNA from damage that leads to cancer.

And they help you stay slim, lowering your odds for obesity-related cancers of the colon, breast, prostate, and more. Loading your plate with produce cuts odds for heart disease and blood vessel problems by 55 percent, says another Harvard School of Public Health report in the *American Journal of Clinical Nutrition*.[14] Feasting on produce can also lower your stroke risk by 26 percent and slash odds for high blood pressure by 24 percent.[15]

The Health Power of 2

Can 2 days a week really change your health for the better? Continuing research focused on part-time dieting says yes. In well-designed studies, women and men of all ages who followed part-time eating plans—some low-carb, others simply low-calorie—saw significant improvements in key indicators such as cholesterol, blood pressure, blood sugar, and the hormones insulin (which helps your body absorb blood sugar) and leptin (which helps control your appetite). Why? Probably for the same reason that part-time dieting helps you lose weight: You can really stick with it, without cheating or getting sidetracked.

Here's more proof that the power of 2 has big health benefits.

♦ **Protection against breast cancer and prostate cancer.** British women lost weight and lowered levels of insulin and leptin enough to reduce their risk for breast cancer by an estimated 40 percent in one study of a 2-day diet plan.[16] And in lab studies, "intermittent calorie reduction" (science-speak for part-time dieting) kept prostate cancer at bay and improved survival times when this cancer did develop.[17]

♦ **Heart-friendly outcomes.** In a small study from the University of Illinois at Chicago, 17 extremely overweight people who followed a part-time diet for 8 weeks saw their total cholesterol levels drop 21 percent, levels of heart-menacing LDL cholesterol fall 25 percent, and triglycerides—an often-overlooked blood fat—fall 32 percent. Their systolic blood pressure (the top number in a blood pressure reading) fell 8 points, too.[18] Improvements like these could lower your risk for a heart attack or stroke by 20 percent or more.[19]

♦ **Dialed-back diabetes risk.** In another British study, blood tests showed part-time dieting improved insulin sensitivity—the ease with which your body processes blood sugar—by 30 percent, while an everyday diet had little benefit.[20] Better insulin sensitivity means lower risk for diabetes. That's important news. It is predicted that by the year 2020, 77 percent of American men and 53 percent of American women will have diabetes or prediabetes, according to Northwestern University researchers.[21] (Today, 62 percent of men and 43 percent of women have prediabetes or full-blown diabetes.)

A bonanza of whole grains. You'll enjoy 2 to 4 daily servings of whole grains—whole grain bread and bagels, satisfying oatmeal, hearty side dishes like quinoa and brown rice—on "simply healthy" days, plus one serving on low-carb days. Whole grains cool inflammation and help control LDL cholesterol. Two or more servings a day reduced deaths from inflammation-related diseases by 30 percent over 17 years in the Iowa Women's Health Study.[22] Meanwhile, the soluble fiber found in grains like oatmeal helps out by lowering levels of LDL cholesterol. It does this by turning into gel in your digestive system, trapping cholesterol-packed digestive fluids called bile acids. They're whisked out of your body instead of being reabsorbed, effectively lowering your cholesterol. People who munched $2^{1}/_{2}$ whole grain servings a day lowered their heart disease risk 21 percent compared with those who rarely had whole grains, say Wake Forest University Medical Center researchers who reviewed seven fiber studies involving 285,000 participants.[23] Meanwhile, 2 servings of fiber-rich whole grains a day also lowers diabetes risk by 21 percent.[24]

OVERCOMING METABOLIC SYNDROME

If you're like most of our test panelists, you're probably fairly healthy. Maybe your cholesterol or blood pressure or blood sugar numbers are creeping up, but they're not yet in a danger zone. Maybe your doctor has suggested it's time to do a little more—clean up your diet, tie on your walking shoes more often—to keep these important health indicators from becoming indicators of health risk. So you may be wondering whether the health benefits of the 2-Day Diet are even relevant for you.

The truth is, they *are*—right now. If you are overweight, are inactive, or have a wide waistline, chances are good you've got a silent, simmering "shadow risk factor" called metabolic syndrome. At least 68 million American women and men have metabolic syndrome by the time they reach midlife. This body chemistry problem quadruples your odds for developing type 2 diabetes,[25] boosts your odds for heart disease by 50 percent and for a stroke by 76 percent,[26] and increases your risk for many types of cancer.

You likely have metabolic syndrome if you have any three of following five warning signs:

■ A waist measurement of 40 inches or more for men and 35 inches or more for women.

■ Triglyceride levels of 150 milligrams per deciliter (mg/dL) or above, or you are taking medication for elevated triglyceride levels.

- HDL, or "good," cholesterol level below 40 mg/dL for men and below 50 mg/dL for women, or you are taking medication for low HDL levels.

- Blood pressure levels of 130/85 or above, or you are taking medication for elevated blood pressure levels.

- Fasting blood sugar levels of 100 mg/dL or above, or you are taking medication for elevated blood glucose levels.

In metabolic syndrome, your body becomes resistant to insulin, the hormone that persuades cells to absorb blood sugar. If cells resist insulin's signals, your body pumps out more insulin to force blood sugar into your cells. This strategy works—but not for good and not without side effects. Diabetes risk rises because your body can't overcome insulin resistance forever. Eventually, insulin-producing cells in your pancreas begin to give out; that's when blood sugar rises into the diabetes danger zone. High insulin also encourages the development of heart disease. And as you'll read in the next section, high levels also encourage cancer.

The answer? This eating plan. When our test panelists started the 2-Day Diet, seven had three or more signs of metabolic syndrome. After 6 weeks, four of the seven no longer fell into the metabolic syndrome category. And those who still had metabolic syndrome had fewer signs and/or saw improvements in their numbers. In other words, they were healthier. Another nine test panelists had one or two warning signs at the start of the program. By the end, all had improved or completely eliminated their risks!

LOWERING CANCER RISK

Eating low-carb just 2 days a week has also been shown in research studies to reduce high levels of two hormones that new science shows increase cancer risk: insulin and leptin. You've already seen how this eating style tames runaway insulin levels and why this is important for cutting risk for diabetes, heart disease, and even dementia. And back in Chapter 2, you discovered the appetite-control hormone leptin and learned how eating low-carb just 2 days a week tamps down the leptin resistance and high leptin levels that so often interfere with weight loss.

Researchers suspect that the hormones leptin and insulin help explain the link between extra pounds and a higher risk for a stunning array of cancers, including cancers of the esophagus, colon and rectum, liver, gallbladder, pancreas, kidney, stomach (in men), prostate, breast, uterus, cervix, and ovary.[27] An overabundance of insulin and leptin, common if you're overweight, also increases odds for cancer recurrence in survivors and for cancers that are more likely to be fatal.

How could hormones best known for corralling blood sugar (insulin's best-known "job") and for shutting off hunger (leptin's claim to fame) drive cancer? It turns out that the hormones in your body are major multitaskers. Like a movie star who does stage shows and TV commercials on the side, these powerful proteins perform dozens of surprising roles that go far beyond the ones they're most famous for.

Take leptin. Beyond telling your brain that you're full, it plays supporting roles in the process of reproduction, in breast milk production in nursing mothers, in cell growth and division, and in how well your muscle cells burn fat for energy. Leptin also seems to play a role in keeping cells sensitive to insulin. Fat cells produce leptin, so if you've got lots of very full fat cells on board—especially visceral fat cells deep in your abdomen—chances are they're working overtime churning out extra leptin. That's trouble!

New research suggests that an overload of leptin stimulates the growth of tumors by turning a protective, tumor-stopping compound called E-cadherin into a tumor enhancer,[28] making cancer grow bigger, faster. High leptin levels also promote the growth of invasive breast cancer.[29] Creepiest of all, leptin helps tumors "kidnap" healthy cells—like immune system cells and cells that normally line your arteries—and makes them develop their own blood vessels (a process called angiogenesis) to fuel tumor growth.[30]

Now consider insulin. If you're overweight, munch lots of saturated fat, and/ or skip exercise, chances are good that your body is resistant to insulin's signals to absorb blood sugar. So your pancreas churns out more and more insulin, forcing cells to let the sugar in. Insulin resistance and high insulin levels are an invisible epidemic in the United States, affecting one in four Americans.

Extra insulin is a cancer helper, encouraging cell growth, cell division, and the spread of cancer cells to new locations in the body. Insulin also discourages cell "suicide"—apoptosis[31]—the body's usual way of knocking off problematic cells. Insulin helps cancer cells become immortal. Excess insulin also revs up a compound called insulin-like growth factor 1 (IGF-1), which fuels cancer in similar ways. High levels of IGF-1 have been linked with breast and prostate tumors. In addition, insulin may increase the stimulating effects of estrogen on breast cancer cells.

In a study from Case Western Reserve University, men with the highest insulin levels were twice as likely to have early signs of colon cancer as men with the lowest levels.[32] In the Women's Health Initiative study, high insulin levels boosted breast cancer risk 2.4 times higher than it was for those with the lowest insulin levels.[33]

When researchers from Toronto's Mount Sinai Hospital tracked 535 breast cancer survivors for 12 to 17 years, they discovered that those with the highest insulin levels were twice as likely to have cancer return and three times more likely to die than those with the lowest levels. Those with the highest leptin levels were 50 percent more likely to have a cancer recurrence or to die—even more than a decade after their first cancer was diagnosed and treated.[34]

Meanwhile, researchers from Temple University's College of Science and Technology in Philadelphia recently found that high leptin levels activate colon cancer stem cells—the cancer cell responsible for tumor development, resistance to cancer treatment, and cancer recurrence.[35]

Does reducing leptin reduce cancer risk? No one's done a long-term human study yet. But in a handful of lab studies, part-time diets (the same kind that lower leptin and insulin in people) reduced the development of breast cancer tumors in animals.[36] British researchers have found that women who followed a low-carb plan 2 days a week saw drops in levels of insulin, leptin, and insulin-like growth factor—results similar to those found in the low-calorie diets that researchers said reduced women's breast cancer risk by 40 percent.[37] Lowering leptin levels is getting serious scientific attention as a way to reduce cancer recurrence in breast cancer survivors, too. When University of Kansas researchers put 34 overweight breast cancer survivors on a diet-and-exercise plan to help prevent a recurrence, leptin was one of the factors they tracked. The women lost more than 10 percent of their body weight and lowered leptin levels 37 percent.[38]

Lowering cancer risk. Protecting your heart. Preventing high blood sugar problems. By themselves, these are all great reasons to eat a healthier diet. Combine these benefits with proven weight loss and you've got a winner—an eating plan that gives you quick results when you look in the mirror plus long-lasting results when it comes to your physical well-being. That's the promise of a plan that combines low-carb and healthy regular-carb eating. That's the promise of the 2-Day Diet. But before we delve into the details of our eating plan, we've got even more slimming, healthy benefits to tell you about, courtesy of the effective, time-saving 2-Day Diet Workout. Read all about them in the next chapter.

Allison Evans

AGE: 43

HEIGHT: 5'3"

POUNDS LOST: 3.8

INCHES LOST: 7.5, including 3.25 inches from her waist and 2 inches from her hips

HEALTH UPGRADE: Her blood pressure dropped, and her "good" HDL cholesterol rose 4 points.

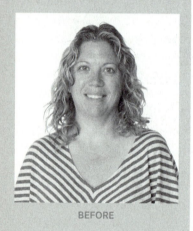

BEFORE

"People Really See the Difference!"

A trained chef, Allison Evans knows plenty about how to make food taste great. But the 2-Day Diet, she tells us, "jump-started healthy eating for me."

"I realized there are good ways to feel full and not-so-good ways to feel full," she says. "If I fill up on high-carbohydrate foods like bread or pasta, I'll be hungry again in an hour. But I learned that if I fill up on lean protein and vegetables and other healthy foods, I stay satisfied for much longer." And that was one of the keys to her success.

A longtime proponent of the 80/20 rule—if you eat healthy 80 percent of the time, you can splurge a little 20 percent of the time—Allison was happy to discover that the 2-Day Diet makes room for that kind of flexibility. "If I really want a great hamburger, I'll have one," she says. "But not a burger and fries. I'll focus on the one food I really want, have the real thing, and then make the rest of my meal healthy. Or I might have mashed potatoes because I really want them. But one serving only— no second helpings!"

Allison missed starchy foods on her low-carb days, but she figured out that a hidden trigger had been inducing her to eat those extra carbs—alcohol. "I like having a glass of wine with dinner sometimes, but I realized that I tend to eat more carbs when I do," she says. She also made another important discovery: "I really like an eating plan like this because it isn't a diet. It's just a better way to eat. I've tried other plans that really restrict carbs all the time, but how can you go through summer, for instance, without having a sweet, juicy, ripe strawberry from the garden or a handful of blueberries with your breakfast? That doesn't work for me!"

Allison's discerning palate was pleased by plenty of 2-Day Diet meals and recipes. "I really liked the Mexican burgers—and all of the recipes with chicken or beef were delicious," she says. "My husband and 5-year-old son also liked the main dishes. I'd add a starch for them or fill up the space on the plate with a big salad. And my son loves eating red pepper and cucumber strips for some extra crunch."

For added flavor, Allison's a fan of searing meats at the start of cooking to create a "crispy, delicious crust on the outside." She also scatters fresh, chopped herbs like parsley or chives over dishes for a burst of extra flavor, color, and aroma.

"I'm planning to keep the weight and inches off, but if I needed to, I'd go back to this diet before trying another," she says. "People really see the difference. My friends are all asking how I did it! I even told my mom and dad about this eating plan."

Already a fan of running and walking, Allison added interval training to her workouts. "It was more challenging than I expected it would be," she says. "I could feel the muscles in my legs working extra hard." She also did toning/strength-training moves at home with free weights. "Keeping my muscles and my bones strong with exercise is important to me," she says. "And there's an added benefit. When I'm exercising regularly, I sleep great."

exercise power:

2 Days to a Leaner, Healthier You

Lace up your sneakers and pull on a comfy T-shirt just 2 days a week—and you'll lose more pounds, more inches, and more body fat than you have with any exercise routine you've tried before.

The slick pitch of a late-night infomercial? No way! That's our promise to you when you try the research-proven, real-world-tested 2-Day Diet Workout. Our exercise plan—developed by personal trainer and walking expert Michele Stanten, a former fitness director for *Prevention* magazine—delivers results in just 2 days a week because it uses the most effective, time-saving (and easy, we promise!) secret weapons around. It combines two secret workout weapons that more and more weight-loss experts say are *the* answer to stubborn, bulging, decidedly *un*healthy excess body fat. What are these weapons?

Secret Workout Weapon #1: Interval Training. You'll alternate between higher-intensity and lower-intensity bouts of exercise as you walk, pedal your exercise bike, swim, jog, or even do faster and slower exercises in the living room while enjoying your favorite TV show. Our interval-training routines take just

30 minutes, start to finish. But you'll get better results than you would on a steady-paced walk that's twice as long, for example, because interval training is proven to burn more calories, blast more fat, and trim more inches than conventional, steady-state exercise routines.

Secret Workout Weapon #2: Strength Training and Toning. Grab your dumbbells and get ready for a quick, effective strength-training routine. Strength—or toning—workouts are essential for reversing the loss of muscle mass that occurs as we get older (starting in our thirties!) and curbing the drop in metabolism that goes with it. In just 15 minutes, twice a week, you'll build more sleek, calorie-burning muscle. As a result, you'll look slimmer and more fit. You'll kick your metabolism into high gear, burning more calories all day long. That makes weight loss and weight maintenance so much easier. You'll feel stronger and more flexible, and you'll enjoy improved balance, too. As a result, everyday activities—from hefting heavy grocery bags to playing with the kids in your life—will be a snap instead of a chore.

WHY CONVENTIONAL EXERCISE *DOESN'T* WORK

We know you've heard all kinds of exercise recommendations by now: Walk a half hour daily. Exercise for an hour most days. Buy a pedometer, clip it to your belt, and log 10,000 steps a day. And don't forget to make time for muscle-building, stretching, and balance moves. Whew! Exercise could become a full-time job all by itself—and who's got time for that?

Don't get us wrong. Moving every day is important for your weight and for your health. Any exercise is better than no exercise. And even steady-pace routines improve health and fitness. Trouble is, most of us don't have time to fit in the 150 minutes a week of physical activity *plus* two weekly strength-training sessions that the government[1] and many health experts recommend as the bare minimum for health and weight control.

If you're not getting much exercise, though, you're not alone. When the Gallup-Healthways Well-Being Index recently asked more than 400,000 Americans about their exercise habits, the project found that just about one in four (27 percent) get 30 minutes of exercise 5 or more days per week. Another 24 percent report that they aim for physical activity three to four times a week. And nearly half move it less than that.[2]

Another problem with conventional exercise prescriptions: They may not really help you lose weight. Take the popular advice to walk 10,000 steps a day. When researchers looked at nine well-designed studies of walkers who used pedometers, they discovered a discouraging fact: People who got in 10,000 steps a day (about 5 miles of walking) lost only about one-tenth of a pound per week.[3] The missing ingredient? Intensity. If you're logging most of your steps while walking the dog, crossing the parking lot at the mall, or strolling around the house or yard, you'll get some benefits—and wearing a pedometer can inspire you to walk more. But unless you pick up the pace (to about 1,000 steps in 10 minutes), losing weight, body fat, and inches will be slow going.

A third shortcoming is that aerobic exercise—like walking, biking, jogging, or swimming—does surprisingly little to help you hold on to muscle mass. It's shocking, but true. Yes, moving your muscles is better than not moving them. But unless you ask them to do a special kind of work—strength- or resistance-training moves—you could exercise most days of the week and still be losing precious muscle mass! We lose 2 percent or more every 10 years beginning in our midthirties. Now, 2 percent may sound like no big deal. But over 20 years—say, from your midthirties to your midfifties—that could lead to a 30-pound fat gain, because with less muscle your body burns fewer calories *all day, every single day.*[4]

The kind of muscle we lose with every passing birthday is called fast-twitch muscle. This is the stuff that gives Olympic-caliber sprinters their speed and explosive power off the starting blocks. It's also the stuff that helps you keep up with the tour guide on that Paris vacation, play with your kids or grandkids in the park, hurry across the parking lot to get to an appointment on time, and stay balanced. When researchers in Sweden and in China looked at muscle samples from younger and older people under their microscopes, they discovered that older people had fewer fast-twitch fibers—and the survivors were smaller and flatter. They just weren't going to work as well.[5] And cardiovascular exercise by itself isn't enough to rebuild lost muscle mass.[6]

Can we overcome the shortcomings of conventional exercise prescriptions and create an effective routine that fights exercise boredom and is easy and adaptable? Yes! Research done with real people—not athletes, not college students, not lab animals or test tubes—pointed the way.

THE SOLUTION: SMARTER MOVES, SHORTER ROUTINES

Now, more and more obesity experts who study real people like us (the kind with sit-down jobs and busy schedules packed with family, friends, and obligations such as grocery shopping, taking the dog to the vet, and caring for kids, grandkids, and aging parents) say the two exercise strategies you'll find in the 2-Day Diet Workout—intervals plus toning—are *the* solution to America's obesity epidemic.

Both are time efficient and effective. You get *better* results in less time than you'd spend on a typical steady-paced routine. You will:

Burn more fat in half the time. In one amazing Australian study, women who did intervals lost *five times more weight* than women who worked out at a steady pace—and they exercised for half the time![7]

Look slimmer and boost your metabolism in 30 minutes a week. Strength training is a time-saver because it delivers important weight-loss benefits in just two 15-minute sessions a week. Twice-weekly strength-training moves, the kind you'll find in this book in Chapter 11, vaporize body fat and can boost your metabolism by 7 to 8 percent. It does this by building more toned, strong, calorie-consuming muscle—but don't worry, you won't look like a bulked-up bodybuilder. Replacing fat with muscle makes you look slimmer. And it helps with weight loss and weight control because pound for pound, muscle burns about three times more calories than body fat round the clock. That means when you have more muscle on board, you'll automatically burn more calories when you exercise and also when you do everything else you do all day—from changing your clothes and walking to your car to sitting at your desk and even just sleeping. Your metabolism is higher. And that can slow, stop, and even reverse age-related weight gain, according to the American College of Sports Medicine.[8]

You may have heard that muscle weighs more than fat. In a sense, that's true. But it's actually a good thing. A chunk of muscle weighs about 20 percent more than the same-size chunk of jiggly, soft, squishy body fat. But that's because muscle is naturally leaner and denser than body fat. It's more compact than body fat, taking up about 20 percent less space. So replacing a pound of fat with a pound of muscle makes you look slimmer and trimmer, something many of our test panelists discovered.

Get a big health bonus. Plenty of new studies show that intervals and toning have another important power: They work together to dramatically reverse changes deep in your cells that raise the risk for diabetes, heart disease, cancer, brittle bones, and more. If you've ever thought there's no way you can exercise enough to get real health benefits, this is important—even lifesaving—news.

Short. Easy. Effective. Powerful. Great reasons to put this exercise plan to work for you. Here's more about why this winning combination works—and delivers proven results to give you the body you want in the time you've got.

The 2-Day Diet Workout, at a Glance

What will you do on the 2-Day Diet Workout? Here's a quick overview:

◆ **Interval training 2 days a week.** Do this 30-minute routine while you walk, ride your exercise bike, swim, or jog or while you do your exercise routine at home. Warm up for 5 minutes, then do a series of short bursts of higher-intensity activity, followed by periods of lower-intensity activity. Cool down for 5 minutes. You set the pace, so this workout is always right for you.

◆ **Toning 2 days a week.** This 15-minute routine uses hand weights that are right for you (you'll find advice on choosing the right weights in Chapter 10). Combination moves save time and work several muscle groups at once for all-over strength training. The plan can be adapted to suit special needs such as back or joint pain.

SECRET WORKOUT WEAPON #1: INTERVAL TRAINING

Going for an interval walk or turning your favorite cardio activity into an interval-training workout will surprise you. Test panelists said shifting from brief bursts of higher-intensity activity (similar to the way you feel climbing stairs or hurrying to get to an important appointment on time) to lower-intensity, slower-paced activity does away with exercise boredom and makes the time fly. It's exhilarating and adds a new challenge to an otherwise uneventful workout—a challenge you control by choosing the intensity level that's right for you.

Compared with steady-pace routines, intervals have been shown in studies to burn fat faster and help exercisers lose more pounds and inches in half the time. In one study,[9] women who did interval exercises on stationary bikes lost 5.5 more pounds of jiggly, subcutaneous fat—the kind just below your skin on your arms, thighs, hips, and abdomen—than those who pedaled at an unchanging pace for twice as long. In one study of overweight men, interval training helped them trim a whopping 44 percent of their abdominal fat, the fat that collects in the torso, settling around your internal organs.[10]

One of our favorite interval studies was done in Australia in 2008. Forty-five women took part in one of three regimens: interval workouts for 20 minutes, steady-pace workouts that lasted for 40 minutes, or no exercise at all. After

15 weeks, the differences were stark. The interval exercisers lost 5.5 pounds of fat—including 3 pounds of abdominal fat. In contrast, the hardworking steady-pace group ended up just like the no-exercise group—both *gained* a pound of body fat! Put another way, intervals let study volunteers shed 11.5 percent of their body fat—and almost 10 percent of their belly fat—while conventional exercise led to a 9.5 percent *increase* in body fat.[11]

The researchers even noted that interval exercisers succeeded in doing something that exercise experts said was impossible: They spot-reduced their legs and torsos a little. Those areas worked the hardest during exercise (study volunteers rode exercise bikes) and seemed to lose a little extra fat and gain a little extra lean muscle—leaving their legs and midsections slimmer and shapelier. Nice!

The Weight-Loss Bonus

Exercising at a steady pace calls on your body's aerobic system, which uses oxygen to burn carbohydrates and fat for energy. By pushing yourself harder for very brief periods of time, you activate your body's anaerobic system, which skips the oxygen and burns pure carbohydrates stored inside muscle cells.

Why do intervals boost weight loss? For one thing, intervals train your body to burn more carbs and more fat during exercise and afterward, research shows.[12] After using up the carbs, called glycogen, inside muscle cells, your body sends in more carbs in the form of blood sugar. Calling on your anaerobic system stimulates the production of more mitochondria—those "power plants" inside muscle cells—so your body can produce more energy and, in the process, burn more fat

Q&A: Frequent Workouts

Q: Is it okay to exercise more than 2 days a week if I want?

A: Of course! If you already walk, take a fitness class, jog, or take part in another fitness activity, keep it up! More exercise is beneficial because you'll burn more calories and further improve cardiovascular fitness. Just be sure to continue your interval-training and toning/strength-building routines so you don't miss out on their important weight-loss and health benefits. You'll learn in Chapter 10 how to use interval training in many other types of activity—without even going to the gym. Just be sure to limit interval workouts to two to three per week; for best results, your body needs a little in-between recovery time.

Reclaim Your Zing!

Ever wonder how the food you eat and the air you breathe get turned into the energy that powers your body and your brain? Thank millions of teeny-tiny power plants in your muscles (there are thousands in every cell!).[13]

You'd need a powerful microscope to see these tube-shaped wonders called mitochondria, but just picture this: Magnified, they look like Good & Plenty candies suspended in a bowl of Jell-O. Each one transforms blood sugar and fatty acids from the food you eat into fuel your body can burn.[14] Having lots of healthy, active mitochondria on board keeps your metabolism high.

Mitochondria sound like something only a science nerd could love. But taking care of them is emerging as an essential step for weight loss and staying healthy. Aging, too much sitting, and overeating zap these little motors, leaving you feeling weak and boosting odds for weight gain, diabetes, heart problems, Alzheimer's disease, cancer, and reduced immunity.[15]

As you'll discover in this chapter, the 2-Day Diet Workout revitalizes these cell-deep energizers. Interval training helps your mitochondria work harder and even helps your body build more (and bigger) mitochondria. In one Canadian study, women who did seven interval-training workouts over 2 weeks also gave their mitochondria a workout; these power plants worked about 30 percent better by the end of the study than they did at the start—burning more fats and glucose (blood sugar).[16] And in a study from the University of Pittsburgh, overweight and inactive people who participated in a 12-week exercise program actually grew more mitochondria—and made the ones they already had larger. Muscle tests showed that mitochondrial volume, which measures number and size together, increased by about 50 percent.[17]

More power plants and better-working power plants—that's the formula for more energy. No wonder our test panelists reported that the 2-Day Diet Workout gave them back their zing and chased away fatigue.

and carbs. Intervals can increase the number of these power factories by 40 to 50 percent in as little as 6 weeks, report researchers from Canada's York University in a study published in the *Journal of Applied Physiology*. Intervals also turbocharge an enzyme involved with fat burning inside mitochondria, say experts at the Pennington Biomedical Research Center in Baton Rouge, Louisiana. So these little power plants work better, too.[18]

The verdict? When Australian interval-training researchers reviewed the evidence in 2011, they concluded that interval training "may be more effective at reducing subcutaneous and abdominal body fat than other types of exercise."[19]

Intervals and Your Health

Interval training pays dividends for your overall health, too. Shedding deep belly fat, growing new mitochondria, and helping your body burn more blood sugar and fatty acids is a surefire recipe for lifelong good health. These health protectors lower your risk for diabetes, heart disease, and more in several important ways:

Less belly fat means less bodywide inflammation. Deep abdominal fat—think of it as vicious, visceral fat—doesn't just store extra fat. It sends out a nasty brew of inflammatory chemicals that mute your body's ability to absorb blood sugar, it encourages the growth of heart-menacing plaque in artery walls, and it boosts your risk for cancer and even for a weaker, more fracture-prone skeleton. Getting rid of belly fat gives your well-being an instant boost.

Tuned-up mitochondria tune out diabetes risk. There's growing evidence that when the power plants in your cells aren't burning sugar and fats efficiently, the risk for blood sugar problems grows.[20, 21] Powering up your personal power plants reverses the risk.[22]

Healthier blood vessels lower blood pressure. It has been found that short

The Workout That Stops Cravings Three Ways

Combining vigorous exercise with strength training—as you will with the 2-Day Diet Workout—doesn't just burn calories and rev your metabolism. It also helps curb cravings and short-circuit hunger pangs. People who do both types of exercise see levels of ghrelin—the "Hey, my stomach's rumbling! Let's eat!" hormone—fall, report researchers from the United Kingdom's Loughborough University.[23] Exercise raises levels of an appetite-suppressing hormone called peptide YY, too, say researchers from Japan[24] and from East Carolina University in Greenville, North Carolina.[25] And Brazilian researchers recently discovered yet another benefit: Exercise of all sorts makes brain cells that help control the urge to eat more sensitive to leptin, your body's "I'm full, time to get up from the table" hormone.[26]

bursts of higher-intensity activity help make stiff arteries more flexible—a benefit that can help keep blood pressure in a healthier range, say researchers from Canada's McMaster University.[27]

Lower leptin levels for less cancer risk. As you discovered in Chapter 2, levels of the appetite-control hormone leptin rise as we put on extra pounds. Leptin can also fuel the growth of cancer cells and may explain the link between obesity and higher risk for several types of cancer. Interval training lowered leptin levels 11 percent in the Australian study described earlier in this chapter.[28]

SECRET WORKOUT WEAPON #2: STRENGTH TRAINING AND TONING

Don't underestimate the power hidden in the combination moves and comfortable weights you'll lift on the 2-Day Diet Workout. In 15 minutes just twice a

The Mystery of the Disappearing Muscle Mass

It's not fair. Scientific studies show that by the time most of us celebrate our 35th birthday, the forces of aging are slowly, steadily, and silently stealing muscle and replacing it with body fat. You can't feel it or see it at first, but this hidden swap slows your metabolism and can lead to weight gain, less of the peppy zing that makes physical activity feel easy, and extra risk for a wide range of health problems.

Why you lose muscle: Your body's ability to build the proteins that replenish muscles dwindles with age. So do levels of hormones that help maintain and build muscle, such as testosterone (in men and women) and growth hor-

mone. Skimping on protein, going on crash diets, and skipping strength training contribute to the loss.

How much disappears: You lose, on average, 4 to 6 pounds of muscle per decade starting in your midthirties. Eating well and strength training can slow or reverse the loss by rebuilding muscle.

Why it matters: Yes, a pound of muscle takes up less room (and jiggles less!) than a pound of fat, but there's more to the story. Each pound of muscle burns about 5 calories per day, while fat burns hardly any. Losing 8 to 12 pounds of muscle in 20 years means your body burns 40 to 60 fewer calories per day—enough to pack on

week—with weights light enough to feel right for you (we'll tell you how to choose in Chapter 10)—you'll be doing something great for your body and your brain!

Strength training is the only way to reverse the age-related loss of muscle mass and drop in metabolism that happens naturally to all of us. By building new muscle, you're saying "no thanks" to the hidden fat-for-muscle swap that starts in our thirties and "yes" to a younger body. Studies show that you can add 3 pounds of lean, calorie-torching muscle in 2½ months of strength training and at the same time lose 3.7 pounds of fat.[29] That's better than simply dropping weight, because muscle is firmer (it takes up 20 percent less space, so you look more trim, fit, and toned) and it burns calories round the clock—when you're walking, working, watching TV, or just sleeping.

Strength training also rebuilds the fast-twitch muscle that goes first as we age.[30] As a result, you can increase your walking speed, which means you'll get more out of every workout and every move you make all day long. In one study,

plenty of extra pounds every year. Experts estimate that in a decade, you could put on an extra 15.6 pounds of body fat.[31]

Less muscle on board makes maintaining and losing weight more difficult. The combination of less muscle and more body fat (especially deep belly fat) also hurts your body's ability to process blood sugar and boosts levels of chronic, bodywide inflammation. Your risk for diabetes, heart disease, high blood pressure, cancer, and even brittle bones goes up.

How to tell if you're losing muscle: You can lose muscle and put on extra fat without being overweight. Warning signs include:

♦ Weight gain even though you're not eating more calories.

♦ Trouble losing weight even though you're dieting.

♦ Walking more slowly than you used to; having less overall stamina than in the past.

♦ Discovering that getting up from a chair or out of the car is a little harder.

♦ Finding that lifting heavy items, like a full grocery bag or a suitcase, is more difficult.

♦ Noticing that your blood sugar has been edging upward over several years.

people who did resistance-training exercises built stronger quadriceps muscles—the long, powerful muscles in the front of your thighs—and increased their walking speed by 15 percent.[32] And strength training fat-proofs your body for the long haul. In an Arizona Cancer Center study that tracked 122 women for 6 years, those who strength-trained regularly were 22 percent less likely to gain weight and fat compared with those who skipped this essential type of exercise.[33]

Strength Training and Your Health

It's simple: More muscle on board means better health all around. Muscle burns most of the blood sugar and fatty acids from the foods you eat. If you've got less and less muscle, and if you move more muscles less and less often, you wind up with an overload of unused fuel—and muscle cells that switch from full-throttle to idle.

As strength-training researcher Wayne Westcott, PhD, CSCS, fitness research

Baker's Dozen:
13 Health Benefits of Toning

Call it toning or strength training or resistance training. By any name, moves that build muscle mass have amazing health benefits. As you gain strength, boost your metabolism, lose body fat, and sail through everyday activities with renewed ease and energy, you also boost your well-being in important ways, according to a recent American College of Sports Medicine report.

- Reduced risk of heart and blood vessel disease
- Decreased resting blood pressure
- Improved cholesterol and triglyceride levels
- Reduced risk of colon cancer
- Better digestion

- Reduced risk of diabetes
- Better blood sugar absorption
- Reduced risk of osteoporosis (brittle, fracture-prone bones)
- Increased bone mineral density

- Reduced risk of low back pain
- Reduced risk of depression
- Better balance and flexibility, reducing risk for falls
- Less joint pain and stiffness[34]

Stand Up!

Sitting down? There's one more move you can do—anytime, anyplace—to turbocharge weight loss and protect your health: *Just stand up.*

Sitting for long periods of time is emerging as a serious threat to well-being, waistlines, and the number on the bathroom scale, even for people who make time for regular exercise.

In one American Cancer Society study, women's death risk was 37 percent higher if they sat for long periods of time, compared with women who sat for less than 3 hours at a time.[35] Australian researchers have linked longer periods of sitting with bigger waists, higher levels of belly fat, more insulin resistance, lower levels of heart-guarding HDL cholesterol, and increases in bodywide inflammation.[36, 37]

What's going on? It turns out that long periods of sitting dial down the activity of a key enzyme called lipoprotein lipase, which orchestrates the way cells pull fat and sugar from your bloodstream. A lack of movement tells these enzymes that your body doesn't need more fuel right now. The good news is that simply standing up breaks the spell, because it works the large muscles in your legs, hips, and buttocks, telling your lipoprotein lipase that it's time to get back to work.

"Getting up and moving every 30 minutes is a good starting point," says Genevieve Healy, PhD, a pioneering inactivity researcher at Australia's University of Queensland. In a study that tracked the movements of office workers, she discovered that people who took more short, low-intensity breaks throughout the day (like walking to the coffeepot in the break room) were slimmer and trimmer and had lower blood sugar than those who rarely got up.[38]

Even short breaks help, as long as you get them regularly throughout the day. "Getting up and moving a little for 1 to 2 minutes is beneficial," says Christine Friedenreich, PhD, a cancer researcher at the University of Calgary who is studying the effects of long-haul sitting on breast cancer risk. "Exercise and physical activity are as important as ever, but the new health message is that taking breaks from sitting matters, too."

---

director at Quincy College and a fitness advisor for *Prevention* magazine, points out in a review article for the American College of Sports Medicine, "Muscles function as the engines of the body."[39] They affect the health of your heart, blood vessels, bones, digestive system, and brain. Among the benefits:

■ **Better insulin sensitivity.** By building more muscle and using it, you can reduce insulin resistance, which is what happens when cells stop listening to the hormone insulin's commands to absorb blood sugar. Insulin sensitivity improved by 30 percent in one Tufts University study of midlife women and men after several months of strength training.[40] This happens for several reasons. Strength training inspires your muscle cells to sip more sugar and fatty acids from your blood; it also reduces bodywide inflammation, which, along with fatty acids, contributes to insulin resistance.

- **A strong heart.** Want to rebalance your cholesterol? Start strength training. When 3,042 people did just that in a Greek study, levels of heart-friendly HDL cholesterol rose while heart-menacing LDLs and triglycerides (another blood fat) fell to healthier levels. That combination is important. Keeping HDLs high is as important as keeping LDLs and triglycerides low for reducing risk for heart disease.[41]

- **Lower blood pressure.** When 1,600 women and men did an easy strength-training program two or three times a week for 10 weeks, blood pressure readings improved. Systolic blood pressure—the top number in a blood pressure reading, measuring the force inside arteries during a heartbeat—fell 3 to 5 points. And diastolic blood pressure—the bottom number, measuring the pressure when blood vessels relax between heartbeats—fell 1.4 to 2.2 points.[42] Those numbers may sound small, but they could save your life. Every 5-point drop in blood pressure reduces risk of stroke by 34 percent and of a heart attack by 21 percent.[43]

TEST PANELIST TIP: *Feeling Overwhelmed? Take It Slow*

"I'm always busy, so learning about a whole new way of eating felt a little overwhelming at first," says Anne Marie York. Her sister, Kathy Rocchetti, who also gave the diet a whirl for our test panel, offered Anne Marie great advice: Slow down!

"Instead of shopping for a whole week's worth of food," Anne Marie says, "I picked one recipe and shopped for that. When you realize how easy it is, you're ready for more. You start playing with one recipe and realize that it's really fun!"

Anne Marie took other small steps—like removing bread and chips from her meals. "I also looked around my kitchen to see what I could cook that would be low-carb that I already had," she says. "Since I always have some grilled steak and chicken in the refrigerator that I make up ahead of time, I paired that with a salad and was good to go."

■ **A fracture-proof frame.** Working your muscles tugs on your skeleton, creating tension that tells your bones to increase their density. Bone loss accelerates in women and men as we age. Staying out in front of this risk now is an investment in a healthier future and could save your independence—or even your life. In one German study of 55 midlife women, those who did strength-training exercises maintained bone density in key areas, including their hips and spine, over 3 years and had less back pain, while those who didn't lost bone and felt back pain increase.[44]

Karen Fazioli

AGE: 44

HEIGHT: 5'3"

POUNDS LOST: Already a slim 151 pounds, Karen lost 0.2 pound of body fat and gained 0.4 pound of lean muscle

INCHES LOST: 2—including 0.5 inch at her waist and 1 inch from her hips

HEALTH UPGRADE: Her LDL cholesterol dropped 9 points, and her triglycerides fell 48 points.

"The Belly Bulge Was Gone in Just 4 Weeks!"

"It was all about the shirts for me," says Karen Fazioli, a Spinning instructor and mother of three. "I felt more comfortable wearing more form-fitting shirts instead of my usual boxy ones after only 4 weeks on the 2-Day Diet." One evening, she pulled out an all-time favorite shirt that she hadn't worn in years—a bright blue, sleeveless, body-skimming top that followed her contours closely—and wore it on a dinner date with her husband. "Finally, I felt like I could wear it again without looking like a middle-aged mom with a muffin top."

Already slim and fit, Karen says that her month on the program delivered its biggest benefits at her waistline—a common trouble spot for women around midlife. "Some days you feel like you have to kind of suck your stomach in to look good in your clothes, but after being on the plan, I could just stand there and button my tops and they would fit like they were truly meant to fit," she says. "The belly bulge was gone in just 4 weeks!"

Karen developed a new consciousness about her favorite foods, too. "It made me more conscientious about what I'm putting in my body," she says. "I hadn't realized there were so many extra carbs in my day. I eat a lot of yogurt, so I've really adjusted the type that I choose. Instead of fruit

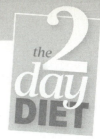

flavors, like black cherry, I'll get plain yogurt now and add a little sweetener and fruit of my own."

The whole family enjoyed the 2-Day Diet meals that Karen prepared. "I'm not a short-order cook for my children," she explains. "I make one meal for everyone. My husband and kids would eat an extra starch, which was the only difference." Everybody loved the 2-Day Diet recipe for Pork Chops with Fresh Sauerkraut. Breakfast smoothies were a big hit, too, as was the steak with blue cheese. "I'm still making the Strawberry Cream Frosties," she notes. "And I discovered almond butter. It's my new favorite—we all love it."

With three busy children—ages 8, 10, and 12—Karen didn't always have a lot of time for cooking. The 2-Day Diet mix-and-match meal charts saved the day. "The charts made coming up with healthy meals simple," she says. "I'm very visual, so having the information set up that way was easy."

Low-carb shirataki noodles were already familiar to Karen. "I've been using them for a while and was happy to see them here," she says. "I'll make some, add cooked vegetables and a little bit of low-fat Laughing Cow cheese, and I've got a great hot lunch that fits the plan. It's kind of a veggie Alfredo, without the calories or carbs."

Interval training was already part of the Spinning classes she teaches, so Karen was happy this concept drives the 2-Day Diet Workout, too. "Intervals are great for fat burning and for building fitness," she says. "And they're not about going as fast as everybody else, but about getting results by increasing *your* intensity, in short bursts, at the level that challenges *you*."

She found that doing harder versions of the strength-training and toning moves in the workout contributed to her success. Her secret? Fit in a few moves during your favorite TV show. "My family laughs because I like reality TV," she says. "But I don't mind. I keep my exercise equipment near the TV and get my routine out of the way while I watch. I'm all about multitasking!"

PART II

The 2-Day Diet

Easy, delicious, and supereffective, the 2-Day Diet focuses on healthy, low-carbohydrate eating for superior weight loss, fat burning, and waist whittling—and delivers big health benefits, too. During this 6-week program, you'll eat low-carb meals every day during Phase 1, the 5-Day Jump Start, then just 2 days a week during Phase 2. On other days, you'll follow a healthy, low-glycemic, regular-carb eating plan for balanced nutrition. The flexibility of choosing your own low-carb days each week—plus the freedom to eat a wide variety of delicious foods on regular-carb days—prevents the boredom, feelings of deprivation, and slipups that derail so many other weight-loss plans.

The details:

PHASE 1: THE 5-DAY JUMP START

- Eat three low-carb meals plus one low-carb snack each day.
- Have 50 grams of carbohydrates or fewer per day. Carb counts average 15 grams per meal and 5 grams per snack.

- Follow our delicious meal plans and easy recipes for breakfast, lunch, dinner, and snacks. You'll develop a repertoire of low-carb meals and dishes you can prepare in a flash in Phase 2. No time? Hate to cook? Eating out? It's okay to substitute the quick low-carb suggestions and dining-out strategies in Chapter 9. Just be sure your daily carb total is 50 grams.

- During the 5-Day Jump Start, follow the 2-Day Diet Workout for best results.

PHASE 2: THE 2-DAY DIET

- Eat low-carb 2 days a week for 5 weeks. Choose the days that work best for you.

- Eat low-glycemic, regular-carb meals the other 5 days a week.

- On low-carb days, aim for a total of 50 grams of carbohydrates or fewer (as you did during the 5-Day Jump Start). Spread your carbs—from vegetables, low-carb bread, fruit, and dairy products—throughout the day; in general, go for an average of 15 grams of carbs at each meal plus 5 grams of carbs for your daily snack.

- On regular-carb days, eat healthy portions of healthy foods—produce, whole grains, lean protein, low-fat or fat-free dairy products, and good fats. There's no need to count calories. Follow the 2-Day Diet meal plans or create your own meals by following our easy guidelines.

- No time? Don't want to follow a recipe? No problem. Use our quick-and-easy meal suggestions and mix-and-match charts to put together the fastest low-carb and regular-carb meals ever.

- Dine in restaurants, grab fast food, or enjoy picnics, parties, and barbecues with confidence. Use our suggestions in Chapter 9 for healthy low-carb and reasonable-carb meals away from home.

- For best results, follow the 2-Day Diet Workout and use the 2-Day Diet journal pages to plan and track meals and exercise.

- Follow Phase 2 for 5 weeks. Our test panelists lost up to 20 pounds and up to 10 inches just from their waistlines on this diet. After Phase 2, maintain your trim new figure and lower body weight by continuing to eat low-carb for 1 or 2 days a week—or by returning to low-carb eating as needed. Keep following the 2-Day Diet Workout to burn calories and maintain muscle density that boosts your metabolism and protects against disease.

Let's get started!

CHAPTER 5

The 2-Day
diet rules

Wondering how the 2-Day Diet plan works? It's easy—just follow the rules! Wondering how to fit the eating plan into your life? That's easy, too. Read on and learn about everything from the best drinks to sip, the best lean proteins to choose, how to work around challenges like food restrictions, and much, much more.

Rule #1: Follow the 5-Day Jump Start closely. You'll eat low-carb at breakfast, lunch, and dinner for the first 5 days of this plan. This helps you get used to low-carb eating, discover how your body responds (for example, if you find that you're always hungry between lunch and dinner, that's the perfect time for your daily snack), and jump-start your weight loss and fat loss. You'll quickly develop a sizable repertoire of easy, low-carb meals that you can use again on any low-carb day during the rest of the plan. That's what several test panelists did when they found favorites on the jump-start menu, such as the Turkey Panini for lunch, the Chocolate-Almond Smoothie for a snack, and the Blue Cheese Steak for a special dinner.

Rule #2: On low-carb days, aim for a daily total of 50 grams of carbohydrates. Spread your carbs evenly throughout the day for optimal satisfaction by having about 15 grams of carbs with each meal, plus 5 grams of carbs in your daily snack. Choose your best days each week to go low-carb during weeks 2 through 6 of the 2-Day Diet—they don't have to be consecutive. Some panelists got their low-carb days over with on Monday and Tuesday; others spread them out or chose new days each week to fit into busy, always changing schedules.

Rule #3: Focus on healthy foods and portion control on regular-carb days. Fill your plate with reasonable-size portions of a wide variety of satisfying, delicious foods—produce, lean protein, good fats like olive oil, nuts, and avocado, as well as whole grains and low-fat dairy—5 days each week. Aim for 350 to 500 calories per meal, plus a snack of up to 300 calories on your regular-carb days.

Rule #4: Fail-proof your plan with a flexible mind-set. There are no slipups on the 2-Day Diet. If you start a low-carb day and then life gets in the way—like a meal away from home where you couldn't control the carbs, an irresistible dessert at an office party, a food choice you didn't realize was higher in carbs until later on—you can simply declare it a regular-carb day and go low-carb tomorrow instead. As long as you fit in 2 low-carb days each week, you're right on plan.

Eliminating the idea of slipups erases one of the biggest mental and emotional causes of derailed diets: the negative reaction that so easily leads to a downward spiral into overeating. If for some reason you fit only 1 low-carb day into your week, just get back on track with 2 days of low-carb eating next week. You could also add a third low-carb day next week—a strategy that worked for some of our test panelists.

ALL ABOUT THE 2-DAY DIET

Designed by registered dietitian Susan McQuillan, the 2-Day Diet meal plans provide all the nutrients your body needs for optimal health. Since low-carb diets minimize grains, most fruit, and some starchy vegetables like potatoes and corn, you'll find larger quantities of protein and fat on low-carb days. On regular-carb days, you'll see more whole grains, more fruit, a wider variety of vegetables, and more dairy on the menu. The combination of low-carb and regular-carb days means you get balanced nutrition—and you never get bored.

Ready to get started? Before you do, check out the answers to our test panelists' most frequently asked questions about the meal plan:

Q: I have a food allergy, food intolerance, or a major food dislike—can I adjust the 2-Day Diet to meet my needs?

A: Absolutely. Whether you are lactose intolerant, gluten intolerant, or allergic to certain foods—or simply dislike certain foods—you can adjust the eating plan so that you'll get all the benefits while sidestepping foods you just don't eat. In fact, many of our test panelists or their spouses or children faced similar food restrictions. They discovered that the 2-Day Diet could be easily adapted to accommodate all of those needs.

Here's how to adjust for common restrictions/limitations/preferences:

If you're lactose intolerant: If you're low on lactase, the enzyme that normally digests the milk sugar lactose, then having milk and other dairy products may cause abdominal pain, bloating, gas, nausea, and diarrhea. Some people with lactose intolerance can have small amounts of milk or products that are naturally lower in lactose, such as yogurt and hard cheeses like Cheddar and Swiss. Others use lactose-free and lactose-reduced milk and milk products, or switch to calcium-fortified soy milk instead. Another option is to take over-the-counter lactase enzyme drops or tablets when consuming milk or dairy products.

If you just don't "do" dairy: Choose soy milk to replace milk in menus. If you don't eat cheese, you can substitute soy cheese in recipes, on sandwiches, and at snack time—look for types with no more than 1 carb per ounce to stay close to the carb counts on your low-carb days. Pick calcium-fortified soy products and choose other plant-based, calcium-rich foods (keep reading for more info) to be sure you meet your daily calcium quotient.

If you're gluten intolerant: If you have celiac disease or a gluten sensitivity, you can follow the 2-Day Diet by choosing gluten-free breads and wraps that are also low in carbs. Aim for 5 *net carbs* per serving. If the label doesn't list net carbs, you can figure it out by subtracting the fiber grams from the total carb grams per serving. And on regular-carb days, just choose gluten-free breads and wraps. The 2-Day Diet contains few processed foods and doesn't rely on bread or pasta to fill you up, so you'll find that many meals are naturally gluten-free. Of course, continue following the gluten-free eating guidelines you're already adhering to. Generally, that means avoiding products that contain wheat, rye, and barley—as well as some specialty grains such as kamut, spelt, bulgur, and semolina—and choosing processed foods specifically labeled "gluten-free." For meals that call for a premade food that contains gluten (like the salad bar pasta salad on Day 3 of Week 1), feel free to substitute another side dish or another meal from the menu that meets your dietary needs.

If you have food allergies: Allergic to nuts, seafood, chicken, pork, or any other food on the diet? Just make substitutions. For meat and seafood allergies, substitute another protein in your main dish. For nut allergies, swap another snack or meal to avoid nuts and nut butters. Test panelists and their families had a wide variety of food allergies, and by following these guidelines, they were able to stick with the plan for great results.

If you dislike certain foods: Don't eat eggs? Never touch sausage? Don't drink soy milk? Make creative substitutions. Find another breakfast, lunch, or dinner that you like, to avoid meals containing a food you don't eat. In recipes and meals, substitute an ingredient you prefer—for example, you can use 1 cup fat-free milk plus $\frac{1}{2}$ cup water in place of the soy milk in the Chocolate-Almond Smoothie. (For details, see recipe on page 112.) Don't eat eggs? Use Egg Beaters or egg whites in place of whole eggs if you must avoid eggs owing to cholesterol concerns. Eat a different breakfast or substitute tofu dishes.

Q: *What can I drink on the 2-Day Diet?*

A: Plain or carbonated water, hot or iced tea—black, green, white, red, or unsweetened herbal teas are all great choices—and coffee are the preferred beverages. Skip sweetened drinks as well as juices. If you love soda, try switching to one diet soda a day. Studies suggest that diet drinks keep your tastebuds "primed" for sweetness, which contributes to cravings.

We recommend that you aim for eight 8-ounce glasses of water per day, adding extra to meet your needs while exercising. Fruit or cucumber water is also a refreshing option and a delicious twist. Just float fruit or cucumber slices in a pitcher of water, refrigerate for a few hours, and enjoy.

Q: *What about alcohol?*

A: One glass of wine or a 12-ounce light beer a day is okay after the 5-Day Jump Start. Beer, wine, and the mixers used in cocktails all contain carbs. On low-carb days, make room for your drink by cutting your snack portion in half. This will keep your daily carb count under 50.

TEST PANELIST TIP: *Try Tofu*

Karen Fazioli is not a fan of eggs, so for a quick, low-carb breakfast, she came up with a new favorite: tofu scrambled with vegetables and a dab of low-fat cheese. "I was thrilled when the dietitian for the 2-Day Diet said that was a good alternative," she says.

To control carbs, skip regular beer and choose light types, which often have just 1 carb (or no carbs at all). Opt for dry wines. The average glass of wine, red or white, contains about 4 grams of carbs. But a dry Pinot Grigio has 3 grams, while a sweeter Riesling has 6. And a dry Petite Syrah or Cabernet Sauvignon has 4 grams of carbs, while a heartier and sweeter Burgundy may have 5. Be choosy about cocktails, too. Although hard liquor has no carbs, mixers do—a small margarita may contain 21 grams of carbs or more. Look for low-carb or zero-carb mixers if you want to enjoy a cocktail.

Skip alcoholic drinks during the 5-Day Jump Start. On those days, we want you to "spend" your carbs on food. But even during Phase 2 of the 2-Day Diet, think twice before enjoying a drink.

Q: If I get hungry, how can I fill up on low-carb days?

A: It's okay to bump up your lean protein servings by adding an ounce or two on low-carb days—especially if you're a larger person or are more active. You can also fill up by eating bigger salads containing leafy greens, topped with a quick, homemade vinaigrette dressing or a store-bought dressing with zero carbs. A cup of salad greens has about 1 to 1.5 grams of carbs.

A big green salad tossed with vinaigrette dressing is a great way to fill up and boost nutrition on both low-carb and regular-carb days. To keep your salads interesting, vary your greens mixtures to include mesclun, arugula, baby spinach leaves, and assorted lettuces. Likewise, think green when it comes to cooked side dishes and include kale, collards, and other greens with meals. A little vinaigrette is great on cooked greens, too. Look for vinaigrette recipes in Chapter 7.

TEST PANELIST TIP: *Love Eggs? Switch to a Substitute*

Many low-carb breakfasts on the 2-Day Diet feature eggs because they're satisfying and low in carbs, and they supply important nutrients such as vision-protecting lutein. But if you're watching your cholesterol, your doctor may have suggested cutting way back on eggs and on full-fat dairy products like cheese. The answer? Nancy Barnes used egg whites for egg dishes and chose low-fat cheeses. "I bought egg whites for frittatas and omelets," she says. "They worked just fine."

Q: There's plenty of meat on low-carb days. How can I avoid unhealthy stuff found in meats—like saturated fat and the sodium and preservatives in cured meats?

A: Choose lean cuts of meat, uncured varieties of ham and bacon, and reduced-sodium varieties of deli meats and cold cuts. Enjoy chicken and turkey without the skin. Fish and seafood are always great choices, too. Some, like salmon, provide satisfying protein plus heart-healthy omega-3 fatty acids.

Leanest cuts of meat include:

■ **Beef:** Round steaks and roasts (eye round, top round, bottom round, or round tip), top loin, top sirloin, chuck shoulder, arm roasts, ground round, and ground sirloin (at least 90 percent lean)

■ **Poultry:** Chicken, turkey, and Cornish hen with no skin (white meat is leaner than dark)

■ **Pork:** Tenderloin, center loin, pork loin, sausage with no more than 1 gram of fat per ounce, and Canadian bacon

■ **Lamb and veal:** Chop or roast

■ **Sandwich meats:** Lean turkey and lean ham

Make your protein even leaner by trimming visible fat and skin before cooking. Don't fry—baking, grilling, roasting, broiling, or steaming are better. Drain away excess fat by putting meat on a rack while cooking.

Q: I don't drink milk or eat dairy products. How can I get plenty of bone-building calcium on both low-carb and regular-carb days?

A: If you don't do dairy at all—or want more calcium on low-carb days and find that dairy products are too high in carbs to fit in—call on plant-based sources. In one study, the bone density of 105 postmenopausal vegan women and 105 nonvegans was identical, so dairy is not necessary for strong bones provided you get enough calcium from other sources. The Vietnamese researchers who conducted the study, published online by the journal *Osteoporosis International,*[1] say the other sources of calcium in a vegan diet may be sufficient, provided you fit them in every day. After all, 4 ounces of tofu or a big serving of steamed collard greens has as much calcium as a glass of milk.

Looking for nondairy sources of calcium? Start with these (and choose low-carb sources on low-carb days):

Calcium—Without Dairy

These foods are good sources of bone-building calcium.

FOOD	AMOUNT	CALCIUM (MG)	CARBS (G)
Blackstrap molasses	2 Tbsp	400	30
Collard greens, cooked	1 cup	357	9
Tofu, processed with calcium sulfate	4 oz	200–330	4
Orange juice, calcium-fortified	8 oz	300	25
Commercial soy yogurt, plain	6 oz	300	22
Turnip greens, cooked	1 cup	249	6
Tempeh	1 cup	215	24
Kale, cooked	1 cup	179	7
Soybeans, cooked	1 cup	175	17
Okra, cooked	1 cup	172	8
Bok choy, cooked	1 cup	158	6
Mustard greens, cooked	1 cup	152	6
Tahini	2 Tbsp	128	8
Soy or rice milk, calcium-fortified, plain	8 oz	100	8
Broccoli, cooked	1 cup	94	12
Almonds	¼ cup	89	7
Almond butter	2 Tbsp	86	6

Q: *How can I find low-carb breads and wraps?*

A: Start by reading the nutrition label to find breads containing between 3 and 5 grams of carbs per serving. If you can't find any in that range, look for a type that's low in calories and high in fiber, then figure out the "net carbs." (Remember the formula? Just subtract the grams of fiber from the grams of carbs and voilà—net carbs.) This number represents the carbs that will affect blood sugar and weight.

Q: *What should I do if I really crave pasta or a sandwich or pizza but want to stick with low-carb eating?*

A: Make creative substitutions for traditional high-carb foods. These substitutes are close to the real thing. Try:

- Shirataki tofu noodles in place of regular pasta. These low-carb noodles are sold in the produce section of the supermarket, with other tofu products.

- Two slices of cucumber instead of two slices of bread to hold sandwich fillings such as tuna salad or chicken salad.

- Cucumber and zucchini rounds as a base for hummus and other spreads, in place of crackers.

- Large, grilled portobello mushrooms as a base for cheese and tomato sauces and other toppings instead of a slice of pizza.

- Steamed or roasted cauliflower mashed with olive oil, sour cream, or yogurt in place of all or half the mashed potatoes you serve as a side dish.

- Lettuce "wraps" in place of flatbreads.

- Shredded crisp lettuce or cabbage as a base for stir-fries in place of rice or noodles.

- Skipping the crust. Try a crustless quiche, baked omelets or frittatas, or baked fruit crisps and crumbles with just a small amount of topping in place of two-crust pies. Or make a crustless pizza by using pizza sauces and seasonings over steak, chicken, or turkey breast or on a mushroom (as mentioned above).

Q: How can I sweeten coffee, tea, yogurt, and other foods without adding lots of carbs?

A: Sweeten naturally. Try stevia, a calorie-free sugar alternative sold under the brand names Truvia, SweetLeaf, and Pure Via. Our test panelists said it tasted great in yogurt with fruit and in coffee and tea.

Q: If I'm not hungry, is it okay to skip the snack or to split it up?

A: Splitting up your snack is a great idea on low-carb days. That way, you can fill up two times in the day when you may be feeling a little between-meal hunger. You don't always have to eat the snack, but remember that it does provide important nutrients—and it keeps you from becoming ravenous. By the way, don't waste between-meal calories on junk food at any time in the diet. Instead, eat small amounts of nuts, nut butters, fruits, vegetables, and cheeses and other dairy or dairy substitutes to tide you over until the next meal and pack more nutrients into your diet.

Q: I'm not a big breakfast eater. Can I skip it?

A: Try to eat something in the morning. Plenty of research shows that breakfast eaters have an easier time losing weight and keeping it off. The good news is that you don't have to eat a full breakfast and you don't have to eat it the minute you wake up. Have part of your breakfast before you leave for work or later in the morning. Have the rest as a snack.

Why does breakfast matter? Nearly 80 percent of participants in the National Weight Control Registry—dieters who've shed at least 30 pounds and kept the weight off for at least 12 months—eat in the morning, report University of Colorado researchers.[2] There's something uniquely satisfying about breakfast that carries you through the day. A University of Texas study of 867 people finds that breakfast eaters consume fewer calories and less fat throughout the day than those who skip breakfast or eat hardly anything.[3]

Eggs, which are featured on low-carb days on the 2-Day Diet, are a great choice. Hard-cooked eggs in their shells keep for up to 7 days in the refrigerator.[4] So boil some in advance and you're ready for the busiest morning. You'll crave-proof your day. When 30 overweight women munched 340 calories' worth of either eggs and toast or bagel and cream cheese, St. Louis University researchers found that the egg group felt more satisfied and less hungry a few hours later. As a result, they ate 140 fewer calories at lunch and 290 fewer calories for the day than the bagel group.[5]

Q: I eat out frequently. How can I stay on a low-carb diet?

A: It's easier than you may think. Our test panelists report that eating out was no problem on the 2-Day Diet, even on low-carb days. Guarantee success by planning to order a meal that's similar to the meals on the menu plan. Or order the basic meal that many test panelists said became their go-to choice when eating away from home: a lean, healthy protein (such as skinless

TEST PANELIST TIP: *Eating Out? Check Carb Counts on Your Smartphone First*

Find a carb-count app for your smartphone. Diane Mann used one while eating out with her family—something they do often, with two daughters involved in after-school and evening activities. "I could always find something to eat," she says. "Carb counts usually aren't shown on menus, but I found them fast with my phone and ordered with confidence."

chicken, broiled/baked fish, or lean beef or pork—without sauces or a crunchy, fried crust) and a big green salad or two nonstarchy vegetables. For more ideas, check our restaurant suggestions in Chapter 9 or go online. Many restaurants now list nutrition information for all offerings on the Internet, letting you choose in advance.

Q: We order a lot of takeout on busy nights when nobody wants to cook. What can I do on low-carb days that's just as fast and easy?

A: Keep an "emergency meal" on hand. Why not keep individually packed boneless, skinless chicken breasts and a bag of lower-carb vegetables such as chopped kale, green beans, or zucchini in the freezer? Defrost and sauté the chicken while the veggies steam; add salad greens, top with a shake of oil, vinegar, and your favorite seasonings—and dinner's ready.

Q: How can I cut down the recipes on the plan so they're enough for one or two people?

A: We suggest cutting the recipe ingredients in half. This will generally provide 2 servings—enough for two people or enough for you to enjoy a meal and have leftovers for tomorrow's lunch or dinner. It's an easy way to cook ahead. You can also freeze a portion to enjoy later on.

Q: I don't really use recipes. Is there an easier way to make meals that are low-carb and regular-carb?

A: Yes. You can follow our mix-and-match chart on pages 200–201 for low-carb and regular-carb meals in a flash. You can also create your own meals and stay within the guidelines using the food options on page 197. These charts list net carbs as well as calories for readers who prefer to count calories on regular-carb days. Remember to keep meals to about 15 grams of carbohydrates on low-carb days and snacks to about 5 grams of carbs. On regular-carb days, keep meals to about 450 to 550 calories and snacks to 150 to 250 calories. Don't want to count calories on regular-carb days? Use the guidelines for recommended food groups and portions, found on page 121.

Renee Guzenski

AGE: 40

HEIGHT: 5'8"

POUNDS LOST: 15.8

INCHES LOST: 13.25, including 4 inches from her hips and 2 inches from her waist

HEALTH UPGRADE: Her triglycerides dropped 38 points, and her LDL cholesterol fell 21 points.

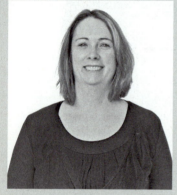

BEFORE

Losing Weight— Even on Vacation

A family vacation at the New Jersey shore in the middle of the 2-Day Diet test panel made Renee Guzenski, an accounting associate at a nature conservancy, a little nervous. Would the temptation of those boardwalk fries and ice-cream cones mean that she'd stop losing weight and start regaining instead? Not if she could help it! She quickly called on the plan's flexibility to come up with a solution that kept her on track even while she was having fun at the beach.

"I decided to have peanut butter on low-carb bread as my breakfast every morning during our trip," she says. "That was so filling that it held me over till lunch. And I did a lot of walking—on the beach and on the boardwalk. When I got home, I just jumped right back into the program."

Renee went through the program with her friend and office mate Sara Phillips, and their buddy system, she insists, made all the difference (read more about their buddy system on page 11).

"It's important to have support," she says. "We ate lunch together and kept each other motivated. Doing the program with a friend made it really fun." It also made it extremely effective. Each woman lost over 15 pounds and more than 15 overall inches—among the most impressive test panelist results.

Support at home helped, too. Renee's husband followed the program along with his wife and lost 15 pounds himself. "He didn't have to lose weight, but he looks even better now. Pants that were getting a little snug now fit him nicely," she reports. "He did it to support me and found out that he really liked the food—like the sirloin burgers and the flank steak."

Renee's own clothes are fitting better, too. "My goal all of last winter was to fit into eight pairs of

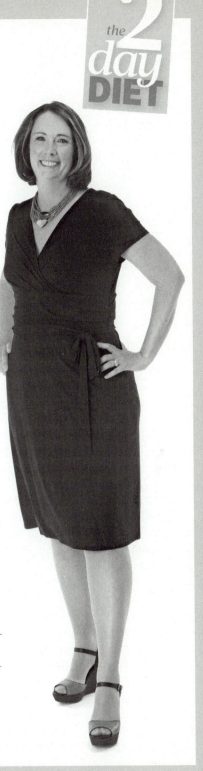

size 14 dress pants I'd bought but could no longer wear," she says. "Now they fit and I'm looking forward to putting them on again in the fall. I'm already back in a pair of jeans that had been skintight before the program started. Now they're loose!"

Other diets she's tried seemed too restrictive, but the 2-Day Diet had lots of choices and plenty of food to keep her full and satisfied. "You can stick with this plan because you get so many options," she says. "It's low-carb just 2 days a week, so you always have a regular-carb day coming up soon. And the food is so good. You can even go out for dinner and not blow it. My husband and I went out to dinner for our wedding anniversary during the plan. I splurged a little on an appetizer, but I didn't have to feel guilty."

One day, she even treated herself to two slices of pizza—and still lost weight. "I actually dropped 2 pounds for that week," she says. And since the plan allows a square of dark chocolate as a dessert treat once in a while, a dark chocolate bunny she'd saved from Easter came in handy. "I'd have just a little and feel really satisfied. I was never hungry."

One splurge that Renee grew to love: nuts and seeds. "Every time I go to the store now, I buy walnuts and almonds, plus sunflower seeds for my husband. We put a few on our salads." Renee has also developed a new appreciation for the natural sweetness of fruit. "I can eat a whole bowl of watermelon," she says. "I loved that there was fruit even on low-carb days. Strawberries, blueberries, cantaloupe, pineapple—they're all on my healthy new shopping list."

CHAPTER 6

Prep for diet success

Weight-loss success goes beyond food and exercise. The right mind-set and smart strategies can boost the amount of weight and body fat you lose—and help you stay satisfied, craving-free, and on track no matter what life throws at you. Make your 2-Day Diet journey a success with these research-proven strategies.

SLOW DOWN FOR MORE SATISFACTION

Eating slowly—by taking small bites, chewing thoroughly, and putting down your fork or spoon between bites—can help you sidestep overeating and still feel full. Research proves it. In a University of Rhode Island study, women ate 66 fewer calories when they were asked to eat a meal slowly than when they were asked to eat as quickly as possible.[1] Stretching out your meal also gives satiety hormones from your digestive system time to act, so you feel fuller. In a Greek study, men had lower levels of these appetite-controlling "gut peptide" hormones in their bloodstream when they wolfed down 10 ounces of ice cream in 5 minutes, but more of them when they made the treat last for 30 minutes.[2]

The Rhode Island researchers also found that eating fast is a bad habit more often linked with being overweight than with having a body weight within a healthy range. Guys: You may need a little extra practice to nail this skill. The same scientists have found that men tend to down 80 calories per minute, compared with 50 per minute for women.[3]

Making healthy food choices can help you eat more slowly. Munching whole grains rather than refined grains (such as brown rice or whole grain bread instead of white rice or white bread) can also help you eat more slowly, say the same University of Rhode Island researchers.

DRINK UP

Never underestimate the power of water. A glass or two before meals helps you feel fuller and can turbocharge your weight loss. In a series of studies, researchers from Virginia Tech found that two 8-ounce glasses of water just before a meal helped dieters eat 75 to 90 fewer calories per meal and lose an extra 5 pounds in 12 weeks, compared with dieters who didn't use this strategy.[4]

Water may even help boost your metabolism.[5] Sipping three 16-ounce glasses a day revs metabolism enough to burn up to an extra 1,400 calories per month, researchers say.[6] Water stimulates the sympathetic nervous system, intensifying a process called thermogenesis, which burns fat and calories as your body works to raise your temperature.

TURN IN A LITTLE EARLIER

Skimping on sleep boosts activation in your brain's appetite center, say researchers from Sweden's Uppsala University.[7] University of Chicago researchers have also found that when dieters get enough sleep—most of us need 7 to 8 hours per night—they lose more fat than when they are sleep-deprived. The study followed 10 overweight women and men, ages 35 to 49. For 2 weeks, they logged 8.5 hours

---

TEST PANELIST TIP: *A Pox on Perfection!*

"Don't feel frustrated if you don't follow the plan exactly at first," says Matt Opatovsky, whose 20-pound weight loss on the 2-Day Diet set a test panelist record. "I didn't, and I still had success. When you start something new that really matters to you, it's easy to feel really gung ho and motivated. When you discover that it involves a new way of eating, you may have setbacks. If you have a moment of weakness or find yourself in a situation where you just can't put together a low-carb meal—like at a party or work event—just recover and get back on track. I had a couple of days that weren't so great, but I kept trying again."

of sleep per night; for another 2 weeks, they got just 5.5 hours of shut-eye nightly. They lost 6.6 pounds during each phase of the study—but the kind of weight they lost was radically different. Well-rested dieters lost 3.1 pounds of fat and 3.3 pounds of "fat-free body mass" such as muscle. But when sleep-deprived, they lost just 1.3 pounds of fat and 5.3 pounds of fat-free body mass. That's a problem, because losing muscle reduces your metabolic rate—you burn fewer calories round the clock, making weight maintenance difficult. Sleep also controlled levels of the hunger hormone ghrelin.[8]

TRACK YOUR SUCCESS

Whether you weigh yourself, measure yourself, or simply notice how well your clothes are fitting, checking in during and after the 2-Day Diet can improve your results and help you maintain. In one study, successful dieters who weighed themselves regularly regained less than half as much weight compared with those who rarely or never put their feet back on the bathroom scale.[9] In another study, 75 percent of successful maintainers weighed themselves at least once a week.[10] It's a great way to pick up on little weight gains so you can reverse them quickly.[11] And that's another built-in advantage of the 2-Day Diet's low-carb days strategy. Once you've finished the program, it becomes a great maintenance tool. You can always add 1 or 2 low-carb days back into your week to maintain your weight or pare off pounds that may have crept back on.

SOOTHE STRESS

You don't need a research study to tell you that it's really easy to reach for food when tension levels rise.[12] Or to know what researchers at University College in London found: Stress snackers don't reach for baby carrots. They head for

---

TEST PANELIST TIP: *Keep Track*

Test panelists Nancy Barnes and Paula Weiant both kept food logs during the 2-Day Diet and say the extra accountability helped them stay on track. "I keep a food log in my iPad," Barnes says. "It's really easy." Weiant had joined a women's running group and used the same log she kept for exercise. That way, she could look back and see the total investment she was making in her health and her weight—and feel inspired to keep going.

Emotional Eating: What Are You Really Hungry For?

Tuning in to hunger, satisfaction, and the experience of eating can help you identify when you're truly hungry and when you may be eating for other reasons. You'll find a hunger/satisfaction rating in the daily journal pages for the 2-Day Diet and 5-Day Jump Start and in extra journal pages at the back of this book. Experts say there are five key ways to tell the difference between emotional eating and real hunger for food.

1. Emotional hunger comes on suddenly. Physical hunger is gradual.
2. Physical hunger is felt below the neck (that growling tummy!). Emotional hunger is felt above the neck (that craving for carrot cake or mint chocolate-chip ice cream).
3. Physical hunger is satisfied with fuel—many types of food will do the trick. Emotional hunger, on the other hand, can be satisfied by just one specific food—at any moment, it might be pizza or a glazed doughnut or a banana split.
4. Emotional hunger demands immediate satisfaction. Physical hunger can usually wait.
5. Physical hunger leaves no guilt behind. Emotional hunger leaves plenty of guilt in its wake.

What if you discover you're craving food but you're not truly hungry? Take a 5-minute break. Relax with one of the stress-reducing strategies outlined on page 80. Then think about what you need emotionally. Do you just need a change of scenery and a chance to stretch tight muscles after spending hours at your desk? Do you need to take care of a problem at home, in an important relationship, or at the office? Are you lonely and need to chat with a friend? Bored? Identifying your true hunger, and feeding it without food, will do more than prevent weight gain. It will make you happier.

high-sugar, high-fat, high-calorie foods (that explains why it's so easy to grab a doughnut and not even notice the bowl of oranges on the kitchen counter when stress soars!).[13] The good news? Practicing stress reduction and mindful eating can stress-proof your diet and help you lose more body fat.

In research from New Zealand that tracked 225 overweight women embarking on healthy-living programs, only those who learned stress management techniques—muscle relaxation and deep breathing—lost weight: 5.5 pounds apiece.[14] And in a new study from the University of California at San Francisco, women

(continued on page 80)

Dale Honig

AGE: 67

HEIGHT: 5'2½"

POUNDS LOST: 12.8 in 6 weeks (*Editor's note: Dale continued with the program and lost a total of 20 pounds after 15 weeks on the plan!*)

INCHES LOST: 14.5, including 9 inches from her waist and 2.5 inches from her hips

HEALTH UPGRADE: She lost 10.8 pounds of body fat; her blood pressure fell to a healthier level, and her LDL cholesterol dropped by 33 points.

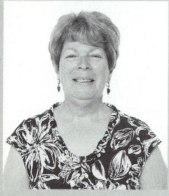

BEFORE

A Sassy New Look

When Dale Honig walked onto the beach in her swimsuit during a vacation with her significant other, he noticed her slim new shape right away. The women in her swim class saw it, too, and so did her hairdresser. "The results were really surprising. I've never lost this much weight and this many inches in such a short period of time," says Dale, who's retired from a marketing position in the long-term care industry. "I've gone to the same hair-dresser for 30 years. He said I looked thinner—he even cut my hair differently because he wanted to give me a more sassy look!"

Though she'd always been slim, Dale says she gained stubborn weight and developed "a puffy look" a few years ago, around the time her doctor told her that her thyroid function was low. "I was hoping this program would help with that, and it did," she notes. "You know how you suck your gut in to get into clothes? I don't have to do that any-more. The waistbands of my pants had to be taken in. My clothes look right on me—nice and smooth. My figure is changing in a good way."

Active in her retirement, Dale belongs to several book groups and goes to a hydrobiking class at her gym 2 days a week. She also walks regularly and rides a road bike on local trails and through her neighborhood. "Thanks to my former job in long-term care, I'm very conscious of the importance of keeping your brain healthy as you get older," she says. "Exercise is important, and so is diet. I was so happy to find that a lot of what experts suggest as the right foods for a healthy brain are in this program—like nuts, berries, whole grains, and good

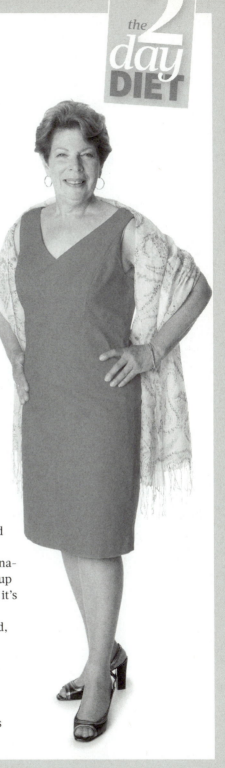

fats. I'm a big supporter of a good, sensible diet to help keep your brain in shape, and on this diet, I found I was eating exactly the right way. It's so positive."

Never a between-meal nibbler, Dale did find portion control at meals challenging on the plan. "I enjoy eating," she says, "so I had to learn not to go back for seconds and thirds—and that was very hard psychologically. I have to stay focused and tell myself when it's time to stop." When she did that, she realized that she felt satisfied with the smaller, healthy portions. "Having 2 ounces of Cheddar cheese and half of an apple as a snack was all I needed," she says. "After a while, it was second nature—as if my stomach had shrunk. I even found that half of a wrap sandwich was plenty for me. I'd take the rest home and save it for another meal."

On the 2-Day Diet, she also found unexpected pleasure in familiar foods served in new ways. "Hummus and cucumber was a delicious combination," she says. "And chicken salad in a lettuce cup works well, too. It's pretty and fills you up—and it's actually very trendy in restaurants these days."

Having a partner to enjoy meals with helped, too. "Every day, Joe would ask. 'What are we having today?'" she says. "Having him as a cheerleader really helped me along. And he dropped a whole pants size, too. He even had to return two pairs of pants to the store yesterday because they were too big. The plan has been great for both of us!"

who weren't dieting, practiced stress-busting techniques, and learned how to eat more mindfully avoided weight gain. Those who reduced stress the most lost deep abdominal fat—the kind that boosts risk for diabetes, heart disease, and even some forms of cancer.[15]

You can soothe stress with a meditative hobby such as knitting or woodworking, by spending time with friends, or by trying simple muscle relaxation or breathing exercises like these:

■ *Soothing breathing exercise:* In a quiet room, sit in a comfortable chair with both feet planted on the floor, your arms relaxed, and your hands in your lap. Now just follow your inhalations and exhalations as you breathe normally—in and out, in and out. If your thoughts wander (and they will—it's only natural!), simply invite your attention to refocus on your breath. As you relax, try deeper breaths—inhale as you count to 4. Let your breath fill your abdomen. Pause for a second, then exhale for a count of 4. Pause for a second, then repeat.

■ *Progressive muscle relaxation:* Sit in a comfortable chair with both feet flat on the floor and your arms relaxed, hands in your lap. Or lie down on the floor or in bed. Pick a time and place where you can be alone for 10 undisturbed minutes. Tense and relax each muscle group in your body, starting with your feet, working your way up your legs, buttocks, tummy, back, shoulders, arms, hands, neck, and face. Tense each group of muscles for about 5 seconds as you inhale, then relax as you exhale. Relax for 10 seconds, then go on to the next set of muscles. When you relax, let go of all the tension at once, so that you feel it flowing from your body. When you've finished, you can repeat the whole routine or focus on areas that still feel especially tense.

CHAPTER 7

Phase 1:
The 5-Day
jump start

Welcome to Phase 1 of the 2-Day Diet! During the 5-Day Jump Start, you'll eat three low-carb meals, plus one snack, each day—getting a jump on the weight-loss and health benefits of low-carb eating. As you immerse yourself in this simple, delicious, and satisfying way of eating, you'll gain experience fitting low-carb meals into your days and develop a repertoire of dishes you'll want to make over and over again throughout the diet and beyond.

Our test panelists and their families loved the tasty, easy-to-prepare 5-Day Jump Start recipes—like a hot Turkey Panini with melted cheese and pesto for lunch, Walnut-Crusted Chicken Breasts with Basil Sauce for dinner, and the Chocolate-Almond Smoothie for a snack. They discovered breakfasts for busy mornings, satisfying lunches and dinners worth lingering over—and strategies for eating-out and for no-time-to-cook days, too. (Although we recommend that you follow the 5-Day Jump Start meal plans, you can use the fast meal and eating-out strategies outlined in Chapter 9 if necessary.)

Many of the low-carb meals featured in the 5-Day Jump Start became favorites that our test panelists kept on making and enjoying during Phase 2 of the 2-Day Diet—and even after their official "diet" ended.

During the 5-Day Jump Start, you will:

1. **Eat low-carb:** You'll follow a set meal and snack plan that totals 50 carbohydrates per day. Each meal has roughly 15 grams of carbs, each snack roughly 5 grams, though numbers may vary.

2. **Move:** You'll start the 2-Day Diet Workout. Choose your days and start reaping the bodywide benefits of this efficient and easy interval workout and strength-training plan. Walk or apply the interval plan to whatever type of aerobic exercise you enjoy, such as riding a bike, swimming, jogging, taking a workout class, exercising at home, or using a treadmill, elliptical trainer, stair-climber, rowing machine, ski machine, or other aerobic-workout machine.

3. **Plan and track:** Use the journal pages in this chapter to plan meals ahead of time and to log what you eat and when you exercise. You'll also find room to track before-meal hunger and after-meal satisfaction to help you notice these important signals more readily. Plus there's a personal tracker where you can note your levels of energy and self-confidence each day.

5-DAY JUMP START MEALS

Developed by a registered dietitian, the 5-Day Jump Start meals are designed to introduce you to a wide range of low-carb meals and snacks, to give your body a head start on the weight-loss and health benefits of this proven way of eating, and to make you a pro at fitting low-carb meals into any situation.

The meal plans spell out exactly what to eat, with step-by-step info about ingredients, recipes, and portion sizes. So it's easy. Check your pantry and refrigerator first for foods you already have on hand. Then take our handy 5-Day Jump Start shopping list to the grocery store a day or two before you begin the program. Stock up on the supplies you'll need and you're good to go. Your mission this week? Just follow directions.

Follow the 5-Day Jump Start meals exactly. Try not to add, subtract, or substitute. For the next 5 days, stick to the set menu, which is carefully designed to give you balanced nutrition while keeping a lid on carbs. The plan features lean protein and good fats, and fits in foods and nutrients that are hard to come by on many low-carb eating plans—like fruit and bread. Watch portions, but don't count calories. The focus here is on healthy low-carb eating.

Of course, if you have food allergies, intolerances, or dislikes, follow the advice in Chapter 5 for making smart substitutions that keep your meal plans low-carb. Several test panelists did just that, with great results.

Don't skip meals—or your snack. Show up for breakfast, lunch, and dinner, and enjoy your daily snack whenever you want. Eating regularly prevents the blood sugar lows and supersize hunger that lead to cravings and overeating. Your body converts carbohydrates into blood sugar, the principal fuel that powers your muscles, your brain, and everything your body does 24/7. Making sure you have a steady supply of this fuel maintains your energy, mental focus, and mood—even on a low-carb plan.

Measure your food. For accuracy, check portion sizes by measuring your food. A kitchen measuring cup and a set of kitchen measuring spoons—not regular silverware or a teacup—are all you need. Using these simple tools will reacquaint you with healthy serving sizes and prevent overeating, which could raise the carb count of your meals. Measure so that your ingredients fill the cup or spoon but don't spill over or heap up; they should be level at the top. (See the Quick & Easy Portion Guide on page 113.)

START THE 2-DAY DIET WORKOUT

Just two 45-minute sessions a week can transform your body. Start reaping the benefits by beginning the workout during the 5-Day Jump Start. If you're extrabusy, you can split each workout into two parts—the 30-minute interval workout and the 15-minute strength-training routine—and do them on different days.

We've penciled you in for workouts on Days 2 and 4 of the 5-Day Jump Start, but you're free to exercise on the best days for you. If you already follow an exercise routine that you like, don't stop. Just apply the concepts behind the 2-Day Diet Workout to your own routine. You'll find all the details in Part III.

Physical activity has benefits beyond burning calories and that keep going 24/7. It helps control cravings and hunger pangs. Strength training builds more muscle so you look leaner and have a higher metabolic rate (muscle burns calories round the clock); helps control blood sugar; makes your body more sensitive to the appetite-regulating hormone leptin; boosts your mood; and helps bring your blood pressure, cholesterol, and triglycerides into a healthier range.

PLAN AHEAD

Many test panelists said that planning ahead was an important key to success. Some planned a week's worth of meals on Sunday night; others planned on Saturday morning before heading to the supermarket. Still others preferred daily planning so they could factor in busy schedules and create moment-to-moment solutions that kept them on track.

We encourage you to plan ahead, too. Start by reading through the 5-Day Jump Start meal plan in this chapter. Make any adaptations you need for dietary restrictions (follow the guidelines in Chapter 5). Then grab the shopping list on pages 88 and 89 and hit the grocery store. But don't stop there. Keep on planning throughout the 5-Day Jump Start. Why not check the next day's meals the night before to find out what you'll be preparing and eating? And how about cooking ahead if you've got a busy day coming up?

TRACK YOUR PROGRESS

Tracking what you eat—and when you eat it—is a time-tested key to weight-loss success. One recent study from Kaiser Permanente's Center for Health Research in Portland, Oregon, tracked 1,685 men and women over 6 months while they followed a weight-loss program. Researchers learned that those who kept a diary almost every day lost twice as much weight as those who didn't![1]

Logging what you eat keeps you accountable to yourself. It's also a great tool that can help you spot situations that are especially challenging, so you can be armed with creative solutions. You may find that you overeat around 3 in the afternoon, during the classic midafternoon slump, or have a tough time saying no to high-carb treats or second helpings at picnics or parties. Revisit Chapter 6 for strategies recommended by experts and used by our test panelists to get past these and many more challenges. And feel free to use the flexibility built into the program to help. For example, you may decide to eat your snack at 3 p.m.—or, if you're feeling hungry more often, split your snack into two minisnacks, with half midmorning and half midafternoon.

Take tracking up a notch by eating mindfully during the 5-Day Jump Start and throughout the 2-Day Diet. Being aware of how hungry you feel before eating and taking note of when you hit that "comfortably full" feeling during a meal are great tools for weight loss and weight maintenance. Mindful eating also involves slowing down and enjoying every bite, every flavor, every pleasurable sensation, as you eat. Research proves that eating mindfully can reduce overeating.

Developing this kind of awareness can also help you spot emotional eating sooner, giving you an early heads-up so you can take other steps to fill emotional needs instead of turning to food. Take advantage of the hunger/fullness scales in the 5-Day Jump Start trackers starting on page 90 to begin developing this important skill.

On a scale of 1 to 10, you'll rate your hunger before meals and your sense of satisfaction when you stop eating. Aim to eat when your hunger is at about a 3 on the scale. Plan to stop when your satisfaction level is about 4 to 5. Here's how the rating system works:

1 = Starving. You may feel shaky, light-headed, or ravenous; when you start to eat, you may have a hard time slowing down.

2 = You may feel a little light-headed and ready to eat anything. You're overly hungry and irritable; you feel that you waited too long to eat.

3 = Mild to moderate hunger. You have physical symptoms of hunger like a growling tummy and have that "I need to eat soon" feeling, but you aren't starving or experiencing any unpleasant symptoms such as a headache, shaking, and so on.

4 = Hunger-free but not craving-free. You're full—well, at least your tummy is full—but you may not feel quite satisfied. Your thoughts are still focused on food. It feels as though your body is done but your mind isn't.

5 = Just right. Your hunger is gone. You feel full but not too full. Your mind is off food, and you're ready to take on the next task. You feel energized. Remember, it takes your mind 20 minutes to register that you're full, so the "just right" sensation at the end of a meal may feel at first as if you stopped eating just a little too soon. Wait 20 minutes and check in with yourself again.

6 = A little more than "just right"—but not by much.

7 = You think you overdid it.

8 = Your tummy feels stretched and uncomfortable. You may feel kind of sluggish and not energized at all.

9 = This is how you may feel after Thanksgiving dinner. You definitely overate and feel very uncomfortable.

10 = You feel completely stuffed.

Diane Mann

AGE: 46

HEIGHT: 5'8"

POUNDS LOST: 13—including 10.4 pounds of body fat

INCHES LOST: 12.5—including 2.25 inches from her waist and 2.5 inches from her hips

HEALTH UPGRADE: Her blood pressure fell to an even healthier level, and her triglycerides dropped from 116 to 48.

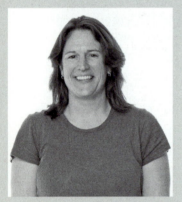

BEFORE

"I Really Couldn't Slip Up!"

As a working mother with two young daughters, Diane Mann knows that keeping things simple and organized lets her accomplish more—even on super-busy days. Her newest accomplishment? A remarkable 13-pound weight loss, made possible by the supersimple 2-Day Diet.

"In the beginning, I had to take the time to really look at carbohydrate counts to understand how to put together low-carb meals that worked for us," she says. "I didn't always follow the menu plans on the 2-Day Diet, but I made sure I ate low-carb at least 2 days a week—and it worked. I used the plan's mix-and-match meal charts and the carbohydrate guidelines and got great results."

Diane didn't just lose 13 pounds. She dropped 10.4 pounds of body fat, which means she held on to a lot of lean, calorie-burning muscle. That's a real benefit that will help her stay stronger, slimmer, and healthier—and will make maintaining her new lower weight easier. Her body fat percentage fell from 40 to 37 percent, bringing her closer to the ideal range for her age. And her body mass index (BMI), a measure that compares her weight to her height, fell from 28.3 to a leaner, healthier 26.4.

Best of all, she did it while working full-time and having fun with her family. A methodical person, she adapted the plan to fit her schedule in several ways. "I really liked the flexibility," she says.

"Instead of choosing 2 formal days a week as my low-carb days, I set out to make every day low-carb, knowing that I'd get off track some of the time and stay on track by eating within the 50 net carb limit on other days. Knowing that I really couldn't slip up—I could just start again the next day—kept me in a positive frame of mind."

Her daughters are involved in after-school activities, so Diane also needed a strategy for quick meals away from home. "We end up eating out a lot," she says. "So I found an app for my smartphone that lets me see the carb counts on restaurant menus. I'd use that when ordering at restaurants and sometimes even when choosing a restaurant. When they serve the bread before a meal, I'd just have a nibble or eat my salad instead. And I'd order an extra serving of vegetables instead of the baked potato or french fries that I would've gotten in the past."

Her snacks also shifted. "Now if I want something sweet, I'll have a spoonful of peanut butter or an apple or some Greek yogurt with strawberries," Diane says. "I used to have cookies or cake and milk at night—one of those things you do when you have young children. Cutting that out is probably one of the reasons I lost 5 pounds in the first week! Amazing!"

5-Day Jump Start

DAIRY/REFRIGERATED

- Blue cheese, ¼ cup
- Cheddar cheese, 8 ounces
- Eggs, 13
- Feta, garlic and herb, 4 ounces
- Half-and-half, 1½ pints
- Mozzarella cheese, part-skim, shredded
- Parmesan cheese, grated, 1 cup
- Ricotta cheese, ½ cup
- Shirataki angel-hair noodles, two (4-ounce) packages (found in the produce section, usually with tofu and other soy products)
- Soy milk, light, unsweetened, ½ gallon
- Swiss cheese, reduced-sodium, 3 ounces
- Yogurt, low-fat, plain, 1¾ cups

MEAT

- Bacon, 1 pound
- Beef, ground, extra-lean, 1 pound
- Beef, top round, 1 pound
- Chicken breasts (4), boneless, skinless (about 1¼ pounds total)
- Pork tenderloin, 1 pound
- Sausage, Italian, sweet or hot, 4 links

FRUIT

- Apple, 1 small
- Blueberries, ¼ cup
- Cantaloupe, 1
- Grapefruit, 1
- Kiwifruit, 1
- Lime, 1
- Raspberries, ½ cup
- Strawberries, 1 pint

VEGETABLES

- Avocado, 1
- Bell peppers, red or green, 2
- Broccoli, 1 head
- Cauliflower, 1 head
- Celery, 1 bunch
- Cilantro, 1 bunch
- Cucumber, 1
- Dill, 1 bunch
- Garlic, 1 head
- Jicama, 1 small
- Lettuce, romaine, 1 head
- Lime, 1
- Onion, 2
- Salad greens, mixed, 5 cups
- Scallions, 1 bunch
- Spinach leaves, baby, 3 cups
- Tomatoes, cherry, 1 pint
- Tomatoes, plum, 2
- Zucchini, 1

DELI

- Chicken, reduced-sodium, sliced, 4–6 ounces
- Coleslaw, small container (4 ounces)
- Ham, reduced-sodium, sliced, 2 ounces
- Turkey, reduced-sodium, sliced, 2 ounces

BREAD, DRY GOODS, CANS, BOTTLES

- Almond butter, 1 small jar
- Almonds, sliced, natural, ½ cup
- Artichokes, marinated, 6 ounces
- Bread, fewer than 5 net grams carbohydrates per slice, 1 loaf
- Chicken broth, light and fat-free, 2 cans (14.5 ounces each)
- Flaxseed, ground
- Olives, kalamata, pitted, 1 jar (4 ounces)
- Olives, pimiento-stuffed, 1 jar (3 ounces)
- Pesto sauce, 1 small jar (3 ounces)
- Tomatoes, stewed, no-salt-added, 1 can (14.5 ounces)
- Tuna, white albacore, reduced-sodium, 2 cans (5 ounces each)
- Walnuts, 1 cup chopped

PANTRY

- Balsamic vinegar
- Basil, dried
- Chili powder
- Cocoa powder, unsweetened
- Mayonnaise
- Mustard, Dijon
- Olive oil
- Oregano, dried
- Pepper
- Rosemary, dried
- Salt
- Vinegar, red wine

5-Day Jump Start

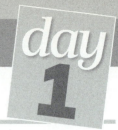

Check what you ate or write in substitutions below.
(Asterisk indicates recipe provided later in chapter)

BREAKFAST *15 GRAMS CARBOHYDRATES*

- ☐ ½ cup low-fat plain yogurt
- ☐ 2 tablespoons blueberries
- ☐ 3 tablespoons natural almonds, finely chopped
- ☐ 2 slices crisp bacon

Per serving: 281 calories, 16 g protein, 15 g carbohydrates, 18 g fat, 4 g saturated fat, 2 g fiber, 456 mg sodium

SUBSTITUTIONS/NOTES:

| RATE YOUR HUNGER BEFORE EATING: | 1 | 2 | 3 | 4 | 5 | 6 | 7 | 8 | 9 | 10 |
| RATE YOUR SATISFACTION AFTERWARD: | 1 | 2 | 3 | 4 | 5 | 6 | 7 | 8 | 9 | 10 |

LUNCH *23 GRAMS CARBOHYDRATES*

- ☐ Turkey Panini*
- ☐ 1 cup mixed green salad
- ☐ Dressing (1 tablespoon oil plus 2 teaspoons red wine vinegar)

Per serving: 477 calories, 32 g protein, 23 g carbohydrates, 30 g fat, 6 g saturated fat, 8 g fiber, 695 mg sodium

SUBSTITUTIONS/NOTES:

| RATE YOUR HUNGER BEFORE EATING: | 1 | 2 | 3 | 4 | 5 | 6 | 7 | 8 | 9 | 10 |
| RATE YOUR SATISFACTION AFTERWARD: | 1 | 2 | 3 | 4 | 5 | 6 | 7 | 8 | 9 | 10 |

EXERCISE

☐ *INTERVAL WORKOUT* ☐ *TONING ROUTINE* ☐ *OTHER EXERCISE*

NOTES ABOUT YOUR EXERCISE TODAY:

_____

_____

_____

_____

_____

_____

DINNER *11 GRAMS CARBOHYDRATES*

	SUBSTITUTIONS/NOTES:
☐ Quick Pork Picadillo*	
☐ ¼ cup Colby Jack cheese, shredded	
Per serving: 333 calories, 31 g protein, 11 g carbohydrates, 17 g fat, 7 g saturated fat, 2 g fiber, 472 mg sodium	

RATE YOUR HUNGER BEFORE EATING:	1	2	3	4	5	6	7	8	9	10
RATE YOUR SATISFACTION AFTERWARD:	1	2	3	4	5	6	7	8	9	10

SNACK *1 GRAM CARBOHYDRATE*

	SUBSTITUTIONS/NOTES:
☐ 2 hard-cooked eggs	
Per serving: 155 calories, 13 g protein, 1 g carbohydrates, 11 g fat, 3 g saturated fat, 0 g fiber, 124 mg sodium	

RATE YOUR HUNGER BEFORE EATING:	1	2	3	4	5	6	7	8	9	10
RATE YOUR SATISFACTION AFTERWARD:	1	2	3	4	5	6	7	8	9	10

Per day: 1,246 calories, 93 g protein, 50 g carbohydrates, 76 g fat, 20 g saturated fat, 12 g fiber, 1,747 mg sodium, 924 mg calcium, 73 IU vitamin D

PERSONAL NOTES

ENERGY LEVEL   1   2   3   4   5   6   7   8   9   10

(Circle one. 1 = "I'm so tired, I can barely move" and 10 = "I've got so much energy, I could dance all night!")

MOOD   1   2   3   4   5   6   7   8   9   10

(Circle one. 1 = "Down, low mood" and 10 = "I'm on top of the world!")

MENTAL FOCUS   1   2   3   4   5   6   7   8   9   10

(Circle one. 1 = "Serious brain fog, hard to concentrate" and 10 = "Mentally sharp, very focused")

SLEEP QUALITY   1   2   3   4   5   6   7   8   9   10

(Circle one. 1 = "I slept very poorly last night" and 10 = "I had a great night's sleep and woke up refreshed and full of energy")

5-Day Jump Start

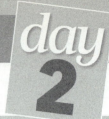

Check what you ate or write in substitutions below.
(Asterisk indicates recipe provided later in chapter)

BREAKFAST *16 GRAMS CARBOHYDRATES*

☐ 2 slices bacon

☐ 2 eggs, scrambled in 1 teaspoon butter

☐ ½ grapefruit

Per serving: 324 calories, 20 g protein, 16 g carbo-hydrates, 20 g fat, 8 g saturated fat, 2 g fiber, 537 mg sodium

SUBSTITUTIONS/NOTES:

| RATE YOUR HUNGER BEFORE EATING: | 1 2 3 4 5 6 7 8 9 10 |
| RATE YOUR SATISFACTION AFTERWARD: | 1 2 3 4 5 6 7 8 9 10 |

LUNCH *15 GRAMS CARBOHYDRATES*

☐ Greek Salad with Tuna and Egg*

☐ ½ slice low-carb toast

Per serving: 470 calories, 35 g protein, 15 g carbo-hydrates, 31 g fat, 7 g saturated fat, 5 g fiber, 1,084 mg sodium

SUBSTITUTIONS/NOTES:

| RATE YOUR HUNGER BEFORE EATING: | 1 2 3 4 5 6 7 8 9 10 |
| RATE YOUR SATISFACTION AFTERWARD: | 1 2 3 4 5 6 7 8 9 10 |

EXERCISE

☐ *INTERVAL WORKOUT*   ☐ *TONING ROUTINE*   ☐ *OTHER EXERCISE*

NOTES ABOUT YOUR EXERCISE TODAY:

_____

_____

_____

_____

_____

_____

DINNER *13 GRAMS CARBOHYDRATES*

☐ Walnut-Crusted Chicken Breasts with Basil Sauce*

☐ ½ cup steamed cauliflower florets, plus

☐ 2 cups zucchini slices sautéed in

☐ 2 teaspoons olive oil

Per serving: 496 calories, 35 g protein, 13 g carbohydrates, 33 g fat, 5 g saturated fat, 4 g fiber, 458 mg sodium

SUBSTITUTIONS/NOTES:

RATE YOUR HUNGER BEFORE EATING:	1	2	3	4	5	6	7	8	9	10
RATE YOUR SATISFACTION AFTERWARD:	1	2	3	4	5	6	7	8	9	10

SNACK *5 GRAMS CARBOHYDRATES*

☐ 1 tablespoon almond butter spread on 1 stalk celery

Per serving: 106 calories, 2 g protein, 5 g carbohydrates, 9 g fat, 1 g saturated fat, 2 g fiber, 128 mg sodium

SUBSTITUTIONS/NOTES:

RATE YOUR HUNGER BEFORE EATING:	1	2	3	4	5	6	7	8	9	10
RATE YOUR SATISFACTION AFTERWARD:	1	2	3	4	5	6	7	8	9	10

Per day: 1,396 calories, 96 g protein, 50 g carbohydrates, 94 g fat, 21 g saturated fat, 12 g fiber, 2,206 mg sodium, 489 mg calcium, 99 IU vitamin D

PERSONAL NOTES

ENERGY LEVEL   1   2   3   4   5   6   7   8   9   10

(Circle one. 1 = "I'm so tired, I can barely move" and 10 = "I've got so much energy, I could dance all night!")

MOOD   1   2   3   4   5   6   7   8   9   10

(Circle one. 1 = "Down, low mood" and 10 = "I'm on top of the world!")

MENTAL FOCUS   1   2   3   4   5   6   7   8   9   10

(Circle one. 1 = "Serious brain fog, hard to concentrate" and 10 = "Mentally sharp, very focused")

SLEEP QUALITY   1   2   3   4   5   6   7   8   9   10

(Circle one. 1 = "I slept very poorly last night" and 10 = "I had a great night's sleep and woke up refreshed and full of energy")

5-Day Jump Start

Check what you ate or write in substitutions below.
(Asterisk indicates recipe provided later in chapter)

BREAKFAST *14 GRAMS CARBOHYDRATES*

☐ Spinach Frittata Muffins*

☐ 2 slices bacon

☐ 1 kiwi

Per serving: 346 calories, 22 g protein, 14 g carbohydrates, 23 g fat, 8 g saturated fat, 3 g fiber,
734 mg sodium

SUBSTITUTIONS/NOTES:

RATE YOUR HUNGER BEFORE EATING:	1	2	3	4	5	6	7	8	9	10
RATE YOUR SATISFACTION AFTERWARD:	1	2	3	4	5	6	7	8	9	10

LUNCH *16 GRAMS CARBOHYDRATES*

☐ 3 ounces sliced chicken (grilled or
roasted)

☐ 1 cup mixed greens topped with

☐ ½ cup ricotta cheese and

☐ ½ cup sliced strawberries and

☐ 3 tablespoons sliced natural almonds

Per serving: 491 calories, 45 g protein, 16 g carbohydrates, 28 g fat, 12 g saturated fat, 5 g fiber,
182 mg sodium

SUBSTITUTIONS/NOTES:

RATE YOUR HUNGER BEFORE EATING:	1	2	3	4	5	6	7	8	9	10
RATE YOUR SATISFACTION AFTERWARD:	1	2	3	4	5	6	7	8	9	10

EXERCISE

☐ *INTERVAL WORKOUT*   ☐ *TONING ROUTINE*   ☐ *OTHER EXERCISE*

NOTES ABOUT YOUR EXERCISE TODAY:

_____

_____

_____

_____

_____

_____

DINNER *11 GRAMS CARBOHYDRATES*

☐ Blue Cheese Steak*

☐ 1 plum tomato, halved and broiled

☐ ½ cup chopped celery and walnut salad (2 tablespoons walnuts) with

☐ 3 tablespoons low-fat plain yogurt and

☐ 1 teaspoon fresh dill

Per serving: 450 calories, 33 g protein, 11 g carbohydrates, 30 g fat, 8 g saturated fat, 3 g fiber, 274 mg sodium
.

SUBSTITUTIONS/NOTES:

RATE YOUR HUNGER BEFORE EATING:	1	2	3	4	5	6	7	8	9	10
RATE YOUR SATISFACTION AFTERWARD:	1	2	3	4	5	6	7	8	9	10

SNACK *9 GRAMS CARBOHYDRATES*

☐ Chocolate-Almond Smoothie*

Per serving: 113 calories, 6 g protein, 9 g carbohydrates, 7 g fat, 1 g saturated fat, 2 g fiber, 125 mg sodium

SUBSTITUTIONS/NOTES:

RATE YOUR HUNGER BEFORE EATING:	1	2	3	4	5	6	7	8	9	10
RATE YOUR SATISFACTION AFTERWARD:	1	2	3	4	5	6	7	8	9	10

Per day: 1,398 calories, 107 g protein, 50 g carbohydrates, 88 g fat, 29 g saturated fat, 12 g fiber, 1,314 mg sodium, 157 IU vitamin D, 1,033 mg calcium

PERSONAL NOTES

ENERGY LEVEL 1 2 3 4 5 6 7 8 9 10

(Circle one. 1 = "I'm so tired, I can barely move" and 10 = "I've got so much energy, I could dance all night!")

MOOD 1 2 3 4 5 6 7 8 9 10

(Circle one. 1 = "Down, low mood" and 10 = "I'm on top of the world!")

MENTAL FOCUS 1 2 3 4 5 6 7 8 9 10

(Circle one. 1 = "Serious brain fog, hard to concentrate" and 10 = "Mentally sharp, very focused")

SLEEP QUALITY 1 2 3 4 5 6 7 8 9 10

(Circle one. 1 = "I slept very poorly last night" and 10 = "I had a great night's sleep and woke up refreshed and full of energy")

5-Day Jump Start

Check what you ate or write in substitutions below.
(Asterisk indicates recipe provided later in chapter)

BREAKFAST *13 GRAMS CARBOHYDRATES*

	SUBSTITUTIONS/NOTES:
☐ ⅛ of a cantaloupe	
☐ 2 ounces lean, reduced-sodium sliced ham	
☐ 1 hard-cooked egg	
☐ ½ slice low-carb toast (3 g carbs)	

Per serving: 212 calories, 18 g protein, 13 g carbohydrates, 8 g fat, 3 g saturated fat, 2 g fiber,
352 mg sodium

RATE YOUR HUNGER BEFORE EATING:	1 2 3 4 5 6 7 8 9 10
RATE YOUR SATISFACTION AFTERWARD:	1 2 3 4 5 6 7 8 9 10

LUNCH *15 GRAMS CARBOHYDRATES*

	SUBSTITUTIONS/NOTES:
☐ Cream of Broccoli Soup with Walnuts*	
☐ 1 cup sliced cucumbers with 1 teaspoon oil, 2 teaspoons vinegar, and a sprig of chopped dill	

Per serving: 321 calories, 10 g protein, 15 g carbohydrates, 26 g fat, 7 g saturated fat, 4 g fiber,
533 mg sodium

RATE YOUR HUNGER BEFORE EATING:	1 2 3 4 5 6 7 8 9 10
RATE YOUR SATISFACTION AFTERWARD:	1 2 3 4 5 6 7 8 9 10

EXERCISE
☐ *INTERVAL WORKOUT* ☐ *TONING ROUTINE* ☐ *OTHER EXERCISE*

NOTES ABOUT YOUR EXERCISE TODAY:

_____

_____

_____

_____

_____

_____

DINNER *14 GRAMS CARBOHYDRATES*

☐ Sausage with Sweet Peppers and Tomatoes*

SUBSTITUTIONS/NOTES:

Per serving: 243 calories, 17 g protein, 14 g carbohydrates, 14 g fat, 1 g saturated fat, 5 g fiber, 619 mg sodium

RATE YOUR HUNGER BEFORE EATING:	1	2	3	4	5	6	7	8	9	10
RATE YOUR SATISFACTION AFTERWARD:	1	2	3	4	5	6	7	8	9	10

SNACK *8 GRAMS CARBOHYDRATES*

☐ 3 ounces Cheddar cheese

☐ 1 small apple, sliced (½ cup)

SUBSTITUTIONS/NOTES:

Per serving: 371 calories, 21 g protein, 8 g carbohydrates, 28 g fat, 18 g saturated fat, 1 g fiber, 529 mg sodium

RATE YOUR HUNGER BEFORE EATING:	1	2	3	4	5	6	7	8	9	10
RATE YOUR SATISFACTION AFTERWARD:	1	2	3	4	5	6	7	8	9	10

Per day: 1,147 calories, 67 g protein, 50 g carbohydrates, 77 g fat, 29 g saturated fat, 13 g fiber, 2,033 mg sodium, 966 mg calcium, 54 IU vitamin D

PERSONAL NOTES

ENERGY LEVEL   1 2 3 4 5 6 7 8 9 10
(Circle one. 1 = "I'm so tired, I can barely move" and 10 = "I've got so much energy, I could dance all night!")

MOOD   1 2 3 4 5 6 7 8 9 10
(Circle one. 1 = "Down, low mood" and 10 = "I'm on top of the world!")

MENTAL FOCUS   1 2 3 4 5 6 7 8 9 10
(Circle one. 1 = "Serious brain fog, hard to concentrate" and 10 = "Mentally sharp, very focused")

SLEEP QUALITY   1 2 3 4 5 6 7 8 9 10
(Circle one. 1 = "I slept very poorly last night" and 10 = "I had a great night's sleep and woke up refreshed and full of energy")

5-Day Jump Start

Check what you ate or write in substitutions below.
(Asterisk indicates recipe provided later in chapter)

BREAKFAST *13 GRAMS CARBOHYDRATES*

☐ Swiss Artichoke Omelet*

☐ 1 slice low-carb toast (3 g carbs)

Per serving: 320 calories, 20 g protein, 13 g carbohydrates, 20 g fat, 7 g saturated fat, 3 g fiber,
265 mg sodium

SUBSTITUTIONS/NOTES:

RATE YOUR HUNGER BEFORE EATING:	1	2	3	4	5	6	7	8	9	10
RATE YOUR SATISFACTION AFTERWARD:	1	2	3	4	5	6	7	8	9	10

LUNCH *16 GRAMS CARBOHYDRATES*

☐ 3 ounces lean, reduced-sodium
sliced ham

☐ 2 ounces reduced-sodium Swiss
cheese (reduced-fat or regular)

☐ ½ cup deli coleslaw

Per serving: 488 calories, 30 protein, 16 carbohydrates, 31 g fat, 14 g saturated fat, 2 g fiber,
628 mg sodium

SUBSTITUTIONS/NOTES:

RATE YOUR HUNGER BEFORE EATING:	1	2	3	4	5	6	7	8	9	10
RATE YOUR SATISFACTION AFTERWARD:	1	2	3	4	5	6	7	8	9	10

EXERCISE

☐ *INTERVAL WORKOUT*   ☐ *TONING ROUTINE*   ☐ *OTHER EXERCISE*

NOTES ABOUT YOUR EXERCISE TODAY:

DINNER *11 GRAMS CARBOHYDRATES*

☐ Taco Burgers and Tex-Mex Salad with Lime Vinaigrette*

Per serving: 487 calories, 27 g protein, 11 g carbohydrates, 38 g fat, 7 g saturated fat, 6 g fiber, 681 mg sodium

SUBSTITUTIONS/NOTES:

RATE YOUR HUNGER BEFORE EATING: 1 2 3 4 5 6 7 8 9 10
RATE YOUR SATISFACTION AFTERWARD: 1 2 3 4 5 6 7 8 9 10

SNACK *10 GRAMS CARBOHYDRATES*

☐ ⅓ cup raspberries with

☐ 3 tablespoons half-and-half

☐ 2 tablespoons sliced natural almonds

Per serving: 146 calories, 4 g protein, 10 g carbohydrates, 11 g fat, 4 g saturated fat, 1 g fiber, 18 mg sodium

SUBSTITUTIONS/NOTES:

RATE YOUR HUNGER BEFORE EATING: 1 2 3 4 5 6 7 8 9 10
RATE YOUR SATISFACTION AFTERWARD: 1 2 3 4 5 6 7 8 9 10

Per day: 1,480 calories, 125 g protein, 50 g carbohydrates, 41 g fat, 12 g saturated fat, 12 g fiber, 2,425 mg sodium, 924 mg calcium, 73 IU vitamin D

PERSONAL NOTES

ENERGY LEVEL   1 2 3 4 5 6 7 8 9 10
(Circle one. 1 = "I'm so tired, I can barely move" and 10 = "I've got so much energy, I could dance all night!")

MOOD   1 2 3 4 5 6 7 8 9 10
(Circle one. 1 = "Down, low mood" and 10 = "I'm on top of the world!")

MENTAL FOCUS   1 2 3 4 5 6 7 8 9 10
(Circle one. 1 = "Serious brain fog, hard to concentrate" and 10 = "Mentally sharp, very focused")

SLEEP QUALITY   1 2 3 4 5 6 7 8 9 10
(Circle one. 1 = "I slept very poorly last night" and 10 = "I had a great night's sleep and woke up refreshed and full of energy")

Shannon Miller

AGE: 43

HEIGHT: 5'1"

POUNDS LOST: 6.6

INCHES LOST: 14, including 2.75 inches from her waist and 2.50 inches from her hips

HEALTH UPGRADE: She needed less insulin to control her blood sugar.

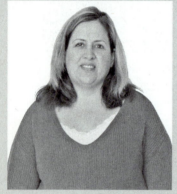

BEFORE

"I Didn't Need All of the Carbs I'd Been Eating"

"I'm more comfortable in my own skin," says Shannon Miller, an accounting manager for a travel agency. "I tend to be my own worst critic when it comes to my weight. But I've lost a lot of inches, my muffin top is going away, and I feel so much better about being out in public. My husband's noticed the changes, too."

Toward the end of her 6 weeks on the program, Shannon spotted a beautiful dress on a sale rack. She loved the black-and-white houndstooth check pattern, the trendy wraparound styling, and the soft fabric. But she worried that the size was wrong—it was one size smaller than her usual. But when she tried it on, she was delighted to find that it was a perfect fit. Shannon brought it along to her final 2-Day Diet weigh-in and photo shoot, where she wowed everyone.

She's wowed her doctor, too. Shannon has type 1 diabetes and counts the carbohydrates in every meal and snack, matching them carefully with the right dose of insulin to keep her blood sugar under control. After determining that the diet plan was healthy for her (it's important to check first with your doctor if you have a chronic health condition), she discovered that following a lower-carb meal plan allowed her to reduce her insulin needs.

"I realized I didn't need all of the carbs I'd been eating. And I realized just how many carbs were in the foods I was eating every day, like granola bars that seem healthy but have almost a meal's worth of carbohydrates," she says.

The mother of two boys, ages 12 and 14, she found an easy way to cook 2-Day Diet meals that pleased

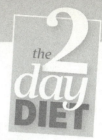

the whole family. "I'd just cut out the carbs everyone else was having, like the pasta or the bread," she says. "Sometimes I'd make extra vegetables for myself. And everyone really liked dishes like the Pork and Apple Sausage for breakfast. Normally my older son doesn't even like sausage, but he told me he really enjoyed that dish and he'd eat it again."

Shannon took on a second job in the evenings around the time she embarked on the 2-Day Diet, leaving little time for formal exercise. Fortunately, her job at a store kept her moving. "We put all the clothes back out on the racks that people had tried on in the dressing room and put all the shoes back on the shelves after people tried them on," she explains. "We were always walking back and forth." One night she wore a pedometer to work to count her steps. The total: 3¹/₂ miles. "That's good exercise," she says.

On Saturday nights, Shannon's family enjoys going out to dinner together. That's when the flexibility in the program really came in handy. "I considered Saturday my day off from dieting," she says. "When we went out, I'd even order french fries—but paired with a healthy main dish now instead of a sandwich. If we went to Applebee's or Red Robin, I'd get a chicken dish. And I never felt like I was messing up the diet, which made getting back to low-carb eating the next day easy. The 2-Day Diet was always simple to follow, and the results were great!"

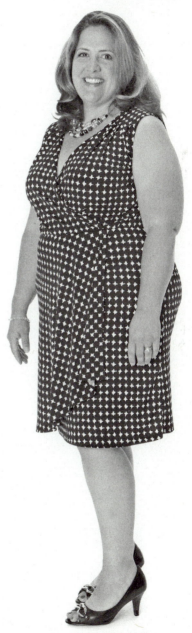

Turkey Panini

An all-time favorite with our test panelists, this panini is delicious and filling.

PREP TIME : 5 MINUTES ■ TOTAL TIME: 10 MINUTES

2 ounces thinly sliced reduced-sodium turkey breast

1 tablespoon pesto

2 thin slices tomato

6 leaves baby spinach or arugula

¼ cup shredded part-skim mozzarella cheese

2 slices low-carbohydrate bread (such as Pepperidge Farm Carb Style)

Layer the turkey breast, pesto, tomato, spinach or arugula, and cheese on 1 slice of bread. Top with the other slice. Place in the broiler or toaster oven to toast bread and melt cheese. (You can leave off the top piece of bread to melt the cheese faster, toast the second slice along with it, then put the slices together and enjoy.)

MAKES 1 SERVING

PER SERVING: 341 calories, 31 g protein, 21 g carbohydrates, 16 g fat, 4 g saturated fat, 7 g fiber, 681 mg sodium

Quick Pork Picadillo

This traditional Cuban hash is usually made with ground meat and served over rice. Our quick and lean low-carb version features cubes of pork tenderloin.

PREP TIME : 15 MINUTES ■ TOTAL TIME: 35 MINUTES

1 tablespoon olive oil

1 onion, finely chopped

1 small green or red bell pepper, finely chopped

3 cloves garlic, finely chopped

1 pound pork tenderloin, cut into ½" cubes

1 cup no-salt-added tomato sauce

¼ cup chopped pimiento-stuffed olives

1 teaspoon dried oregano

½ teaspoon salt

1. Heat the oil in a large skillet over medium heat. Add the onion and cook for 5 minutes. Add the pepper and garlic and cook, stirring occasionally, for 5 minutes.

2. Add the pork to the skillet. Cook, stirring often, for 5 minutes or until the pork is browned.

3. Stir in the tomato sauce, olives, oregano, and salt. Simmer for 5 minutes, or until the mixture is hot and the pork cubes are no longer pink in the center.

MAKES 4 SERVINGS

PER SERVING: 227 calories, 26 g protein, 12 g carbohydrates, 9 g fat, 2 g saturated fat, 2 g fiber, 496 mg sodium

Spinach Frittata Muffins

If you are using a 12-cup muffin pan, spray and fill only 8 of the cups. Use a large spoon to lift the baked muffins from the pan. Gently reheat leftovers in a microwave oven.

PREP TIME: 10 MINUTES ■ TOTAL TIME: 30 MINUTES

2 teaspoons olive oil

1 small onion, finely chopped

2 cups flat-leaf spinach, finely chopped

6 eggs

½ cup ricotta cheese

¼ cup grated Parmesan cheese

1 tablespoon chopped fresh dill or 1 teaspoon dried and crumbled

¼ teaspoon salt

1. Preheat the oven to 350°F. Lightly coat an 8-cup muffin pan with cooking spray.

2. Heat the oil in a small skillet over medium heat. Add the onion and cook for 5 minutes. Add the spinach and cook for 1 minute, or until just wilted. Remove from heat.

3. In a medium bowl, combine the eggs, ricotta cheese, Parmesan cheese, dill, and salt. Add the onion-spinach mixture and combine. Spoon about ⅓ cup of the mixture into each of the muffin cups.

4. Bake for 15 to 20 minutes, or until a wooden pick inserted in the center of one muffin comes out clean. Cool the muffins on a rack for 1 minute before removing them from the pan and serving.

MAKES 4 SERVINGS (8 MUFFINS)

PER SERVING: 225 calories, 16 g protein, 4 g carbohydrates, 16 g fat, 6 g saturated fat, 1 g fiber, 395 mg sodium

Greek Salad with Tuna and Egg

A big salad bursting with Mediterranean flavors—for just 366 calories and 8 grams of carbs!

PREP TIME: 10 MINUTES ▪ TOTAL TIME: 10 MINUTES

4 cups shredded romaine lettuce

2 cups cherry tomatoes, halved

1 cup sliced cucumber

Greek Vinaigrette (recipe follows)

2 cans (5 ounces each) reduced-sodium albacore tuna

4 hard-cooked eggs, halved

½ cup pitted kalamata olives, chopped

4 ounces garlic-and-herb feta cheese

1. In a large bowl, combine the lettuce, tomatoes, and cucumber. Set aside.

2. Toss the salad with the dressing and arrange on 4 plates.

3. Top each plate with the tuna, eggs, olives, and cheese.

Greek Vinaigrette

2 tablespoons olive oil

1 tablespoon red wine vinegar

½ teaspoon dried oregano, crumbled

In a small bowl, whisk together the oil, vinegar, and oregano.

MAKES 4 SERVINGS

PER SERVING: 366 calories, 34 g protein, 8 g carbohydrates, 23 g fat, 7 g saturated fat, 2 g fiber, 625 mg sodium

Walnut-Crusted Chicken Breasts with Basil Sauce

You can substitute almonds for the walnuts and turkey tenders for the chicken breasts.

PREP TIME: 15 MINUTES ■ TOTAL TIME: 35 MINUTES

½ cup walnuts

1 egg

¼ teaspoon salt

4 boneless, skinless chicken breasts
(5 ounces each, or about 1¼
pounds total)

½ cup low-fat plain yogurt

¼ cup mayonnaise

½ teaspoon dried basil, crumbled

1. Preheat the oven to 375°F. Coat a baking sheet with cooking spray.

2. Grind the walnuts in a food processor, then spread on a flat dinner plate.

3. Beat the egg and salt in a shallow bowl. Dip the chicken breasts in the egg and then in the ground walnuts to lightly coat on both sides. Place on the baking sheet.

4. Bake, turning once, for 15 to 20 minutes, or until a thermometer inserted in the thickest portion registers 165°F and the juices run clear.

5. In a small bowl, combine the yogurt, mayonnaise, and basil. Serve with the chicken.

MAKES 4 SERVINGS

PER SERVING: 389 calories, 35 g protein, 4 g carbohydrates, 24 g fat, 3 g saturated fat, 1 g fiber, 355 mg sodium

Blue Cheese Steak

Good enough for special occasion dinners or Sunday night suppers, this hearty steak dish cooks in a flash.

PREP TIME: 10 MINUTES ■ TOTAL TIME: 50 MINUTES

1 pound top round steak
Rosemary Balsamic Vinaigrette (recipe follows)

½ cup low-fat plain yogurt
¼ cup crumbled blue cheese

1. Place the steak in a container or bowl and pour the vinaigrette over it. Cover the container and let marinate for 30 minutes at room temperature or 1 hour in the refrigerator.
2. In a small bowl, combine the yogurt and blue cheese.
3. Heat the broiler. Broil the steak to desired doneness (about 4 to 5 minutes per side for medium-rare). Remove and slice.
4. Arrange the steak on a serving platter, drizzle with the blue cheese sauce, and serve.

Rosemary Balsamic Vinaigrette

2 tablespoons olive oil
1 tablespoon balsamic vinegar

1 teaspoon dried mustard
½ teaspoon dried rosemary, crumbled

In a small bowl, whisk together the oil, vinegar, mustard, and rosemary.

MAKES 4 SERVINGS

PER SERVING: 313 calories, 28 g protein, 3 g carbohydrates, 15 g fat, 5 g saturated fat, 0 g fiber, 208 mg sodium

Cream of Broccoli Soup
with Walnuts

This simple and delicious soup can be made creamier by pureeing in a blender after cooking.

PREP TIME: 10 MINUTES ■ TOTAL TIME: 30 MINUTES

½ cup walnuts

1 tablespoon olive oil

1 onion, finely chopped

2 cloves garlic, finely chopped

2 cans (14.5 ounces each) fat-free reduced-sodium chicken broth

4 cups broccoli florets, finely chopped

1 cup half-and-half

¼ cup grated Parmesan cheese

1. Pulse the walnuts in a food processor until finely chopped. Set aside.

2. Heat the oil in a skillet over medium heat. Add the onion and garlic and sauté for 3 to 5 minutes, or until soft.

3. In a medium saucepan, heat the chicken broth to a simmer, then add the onion mixture and broccoli florets. Simmer for 10 minutes, or until the broccoli is tender.

4. Stir in the half-and-half and simmer for 5 minutes.

5. Serve topped with the walnuts and cheese.

MAKES 4 SERVINGS (6 CUPS)

PER SERVING: 262 calories, 9 g protein, 12 g carbohydrates, 22 g fat, 7 g saturated fat, 4 g fiber, 530 mg sodium

Sausage with Sweet Peppers and Tomatoes

Shirataki noodles, found in health food stores and most large supermarkets, stand in for regular pasta in this recipe because they are so much lower in carbs, calories, and sodium.

PREP TIME: 10 MINUTES ■ TOTAL TIME: 40 MINUTES

1 tablespoon olive oil

1 onion, thinly sliced

1 green or red bell pepper, thinly sliced

4 Italian turkey sausage links, sliced

1 can (14.5 ounces) no-salt-added stewed tomatoes

2 packages (4 ounces each) shirataki spaghetti (8 ounces after draining), drained and rinsed

¼ cup grated Parmesan cheese

1. Heat the oil in a large skillet over medium heat. Add the onion and cook for 5 minutes. Add the pepper and cook, stirring occasionally, for 5 minutes. Push the vegetables to the outer edges of the skillet.

2. Add the sausage slices to the skillet. Cook for 2 minutes, or until browned. Stir the sausages and cook for 2 minutes. Add the tomatoes and stir the sausages and vegetables together. Cover and cook for 2 to 3 minutes, or until the sausages are fully cooked and the mixture is heated through.

3. Prepare the shirataki noodles according to package directions. Divide among 4 plates, top with the sausage mixture, and sprinkle evenly with the cheese. Serve immediately.

MAKES 4 SERVINGS

PER SERVING: 243 calories, 17 g protein, 14 g carbohydrates, 14 g fat, 1 g saturated fat, 5 g fiber, 619 mg sodium

Swiss Artichoke Omelet

This is a hearty and delicious breakfast that you can also enjoy at lunch or dinner on a low-carb day.

PREP TIME: 10 MINUTES ■ TOTAL TIME: 30 MINUTES

1 jar (6 ounces) marinated artichokes, drained

3 ounces grated or finely chopped reduced-sodium Swiss cheese

6 eggs

¼ cup low-fat plain yogurt

2 teaspoons Dijon mustard

1 plum tomato, finely chopped

1. Preheat oven to 350°F. Lightly grease a 9" pie pan with olive or canola oil.

2. Arrange the artichokes in the pie pan and cover evenly with the cheese.

3. In a large bowl, beat the eggs, yogurt, and mustard. Gently pour the mixture into the pie pan.

4. Bake for 20 minutes. Garnish with the chopped tomato and serve.

MAKES 4 SERVINGS

PER SERVING: 259 calories, 16 g protein, 5 g carbohydrates, 19 g fat, 7 g saturated fat, 2 g fiber, 265 mg sodium

Taco Burgers and Tex-Mex Salad with Lime Vinaigrette

When you experience the combination of a warm, juicy beef burger served on a cool, crisp bed of salad, you won't miss the bun.

PREP TIME: 20 MINUTES ■ TOTAL TIME: 25 MINUTES

Burgers

1 pound extra-lean ground beef

4 scallions, finely chopped

½ cup finely chopped cilantro

1½ teaspoons chili powder

½ teaspoon salt

Salad

4 cups mixed greens

2 plum tomatoes, finely chopped

1 cup thinly sliced jicama

Lime Vinaigrette (recipe follows)

1 avocado, diced

1. *To make the burgers:* Preheat the broiler. Coat a broiler pan with cooking spray.

2. In a large bowl, combine the beef, scallions, cilantro, chili powder, and salt. Mix well. Shape into 4 patties and place on the broiler pan. Broil 4" from the heat source, turning once, for 5 to 6 minutes, or until a thermometer inserted in the center registers 160°F and the meat is no longer pink.

3. *To make the salad:* In a large bowl, combine the greens, tomatoes, and jicama. Toss the salad with the vinaigrette and divide among 4 plates.

4. Top with the burgers and avocado and serve.

Lime Vinaigrette

2 tablespoons olive oil

1 tablespoon lime juice

⅛ teaspoon salt

In a small bowl, whisk together the oil, lime juice, and salt. Set aside until ready to use.

MAKES 4 SERVINGS

PER SERVING: 487 calories, 27 g protein, 11 g carbohydrates, 38 g fat, 7 g saturated fat, 6 g fiber, 681 mg sodium

Chocolate-Almond Smoothie

Our test panelists and their families—especially kids—loved this delicious and healthy snack. Choose "light" soy milk and sweeten it with stevia for a total of 6 grams of carbohydrates per cup. That is half the amount of carbohydrates in a cup of fat-free milk.

PREP TIME: 6 MINUTES ■ TOTAL TIME: 7 MINUTES

1½ cups plain light soy milk, sweetened with stevia

1 teaspoon ground flaxseed or white chia seeds

1 tablespoon almond butter

1½ teaspoons unsweetened cocoa powder

Ice cubes (optional)

1. In a blender, combine the soy milk, flaxseed or chia seeds, almond butter, and cocoa powder. Blend on the highest setting for 30 seconds. Let stand for 5 minutes.

2. Blend again on the highest setting for 30 seconds, or until smooth and frothy. Pour into medium-tall glasses over ice (if using) and serve.

MAKES 2 SERVINGS

PER SERVING: 113 calories, 6 g protein, 9 g carbohydrates, 7 g fat, 1 g saturated fat, 2 g fiber, 125 mg sodium

Quick & Easy Portion Guide

Measuring portions with measuring cups and measuring spoons is a great way to recalibrate your sense of healthy serving sizes and banish the "portion distortion" that contributes to weight gain. But most of us will never carry around measuring tools or use them every time we make a simple meal at home. Train your eyes to spot a proper portion by keeping in mind these comparisons to everyday objects:

Portion	Looks Like
3 ounces of cooked meat	Deck of cards, palm of your hand
1 medium piece of fruit	Tennis ball
1 ounce of cheese	Tube of lipstick
1 cup	Closed fist
½ cup	Computer mouse, half of a baseball
¼ cup	Half of a tennis ball
1 tablespoon	Half of a golf ball, tip of your thumb (from top knuckle up)

Anne Morris

AGE: 67

HEIGHT: 5'5"

POUNDS LOST: 16.8

INCHES LOST: 14.5, including 2.75 inches from her hips and 2.5 inches from her waist

HEALTH UPGRADE: Lower blood sugar, lower blood pressure, and her triglycerides fell from a high 282 to a healthy 127.

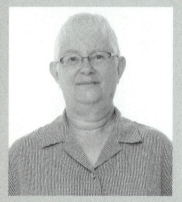

BEFORE

"I'm Stunned at How Quickly the Weight Came Off!"

For Anne Morris, there's a difference between knowing how to lose weight and actually losing weight. And on the 2-Day Diet, she moved quickly from "knowing" to "doing." "I discovered portions on this plan," she says with a smile. "Of course, I've known that it's important to eat healthy serving sizes all my life, but that's not the same as actually doing it. Now I am. Along with low-carb eating 2 days a week, it's really working!"

Looking for fast and easy meals that didn't require a lot of cooking, Anne admits she "dropped the official recipes" after her first week on the plan. Instead, she went with easy combinations on low-carb days—the types of meals you'll find in our mix-and-match chart in Chapter 9. Dinner on low-carb days was something "easy and healthy," such as roast chicken and a big salad. Breakfast was often turkey bacon and two eggs. On regular-carb days, she'd enjoy oatmeal with blueberries and soy milk.

She also found that 6 ounces of plain, fat-free Greek yogurt sweetened with stevia tastes great.

A self-confessed "nibbler," Anne was surprised by how full and satisfied she felt on the 2-Day Diet—she no longer felt the need to reach for a treat. "I used to nibble a lot after dinner," she says. "Roasted soy nuts were a favorite. They're healthy, but they added a lot of calories to my day and to my waistline. On the plan, I found that sometimes I still felt like having an extra snack at night, but it was just an old habit—I didn't *need* to nibble anymore. And I don't need to overeat at meals. If I just wait a few minutes for my brain to register what I've eaten, I'll feel satisfied."

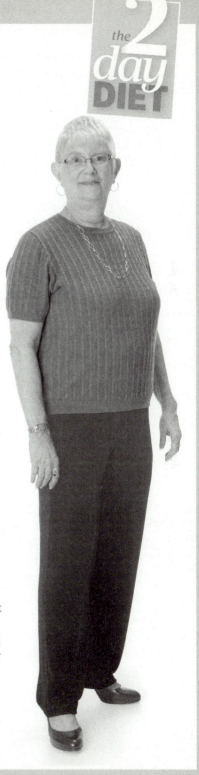

Anne made some important discoveries about herself that will help her maintain her new weight. "A while ago, I started putting on weight. When I got past 170, I felt like I was outside my body, just watching. I didn't take really good care of myself in terms of my food choices. When I got to 196 pounds, I just felt terrible. I knew I had to do something."

One important motivation: health. "I'm working on a family health history so I can pass along information about our health risks to my children—and they can pass it along to their children," she says. "I've found out that a syndrome that makes fat accumulate in the liver runs in our family. That's important to know about—and to reverse." Fat in the liver boosts risk for diabetes, among other health conditions. Fortunately, a healthy diet, exercise, and weight loss can help "slim down" a fatty liver.

Anne also discovered that she's carb sensitive. "If I eat too many carbs—especially refined carbs—I just can't stop eating them. I never feel full and I crave them," she says. "If I start eating bread and butter, I could keep on eating it and make a whole meal out of it, but never feel satisfied. I need to treat carbs almost as a poison and stay away from comfort foods like chocolate pudding, potato chips, and ice cream. I've learned that there are so many other healthy, delicious, satisfying, low-carb foods to eat instead. I just had to learn to give them a chance."

The result? Although the official 2-Day Diet test panel has ended, Anne says she plans to keep on eating low-carb 2 days a week. "Tuesdays and Thursdays will always be low-carb days for me," she says.

CHAPTER 8

Phase 2:
the
2-day diet

In Phase 2 of the 2-Day Diet, you'll eat low-carb 2 days a week. What happens on the other 5 days of each week? You'll simply follow a regular-carb eating plan that delivers a nutritionally balanced, portion-controlled combination of lean protein, fruits and vegetables, whole grains, dairy products, and good fats. When do you eat low-carb and when do you eat regular-carb? That's up to you. Choose any 2 days each week as your low-carb days. These days don't have to be consecutive, and you can designate different days each week.

Low-carb eating is now familiar to you, thanks to your 5-day "immersion" in this smart way of eating during the 5-Day Jump Start. Now, in Phase 2, you'll find new menus, new meal plans, and new low-carb recipes, but feel free to go back and repeat any favorite meals or dishes that you enjoyed during the jump start. You can also follow our easy no-cook and quick-cook suggestions for eating at home and eating out, found in Chapter 9.

Ready to pick up your knife and fork? Read the details, then dig in!

PHASE 2 GUIDELINES

You'll enjoy a wider range of foods in Phase 2. And you'll experience how the 2-Day Diet's innovative combination of low-carb eating and low-glycemic regular-carb eating allows you to lose more weight and inches, burn more fat, and maintain more muscle. The plan's freedom and flexibility make this a no-slip, can't-fail weight-loss plan you can stick to with ease, no matter what life throws at you.

Just follow these simple guidelines.

#1: Choose 2 days each week to eat low-carb.

Pick the days that work best for you. They don't have to be consecutive, and you can choose different days each week so that the plan flexes with your schedule. Some of our test panelists made low-carb "the rule" on Mondays and Tuesdays; others moved their days around. If you start a low-carb day and find that something gets in the way (the boss orders pizza, your husband decides to make pancakes for breakfast, or you simply make a high-carb choice for any reason at all), no problem. Just designate another day as one of your low-carb days.

#2: Choose 5 days each week to eat regular-carb.

No need to count calories (unless you want to). Just enjoy moderate-size portions of healthy foods such as fruit, vegetables, whole grains, lean protein, good fats, and low-fat or fat-free dairy. There's even room for treats like pasta, chocolate, and frozen yogurt.

#3: Be flexible.

If you start a low-carb day but find you overdo the carbs at some point in the day—because you didn't have a low-carb choice at a meal or couldn't resist a higher-carb food—just breathe a sigh of relief. You haven't fallen off the wagon, failed, or even slipped up. Just declare it a regular-carb day and finish your meals and snacks using the guidelines for regular-carb eating (see page 121), then pick another day to go low-carb this week. If you've reached the end of the week, you can—if you like—make up a missed low-carb day by eating low-carb 3 days in the coming week. It's that simple.

#4: Don't skip meals or your snack.

As you did during the 5-Day Jump Start, show up for every meal and snack on low-carb days during Phase 2 of the 2-Day Diet. Giving your body and your brain a steady supply of carbs—the favored fuel of muscle cells and of brain cells—will keep your physical and mental energy high. Eating regularly also ensures a steady supply of the lean protein, fat, fiber, and nutrients that work together to help you stay full and promote good health and healthy weight loss.

#5: Always measure your portions.

Use measuring cups and measuring spoons. If you've gotten good at eyeballing portions, do that. (Refer to our "Quick & Easy Portion Guide" on page 113 for a refresher.) Sticking with healthy portion sizes *every day*—on low-carb and regular-carb days—means there's no need to count calories on the 2-Day Diet.

#6: Move.

Keep following the 2-Day Diet Workout. Choose your days and keep on racking up the calorie-burning, muscle-building benefits. If you're just starting the workout program, it's good to know that you get big returns on a 45-minute investment of time twice a week. The plan's efficient, fat-burning interval-training routine takes just 30 minutes. You can do it while you walk or apply the interval plan concept to whatever type of aerobic exercise you enjoy. The 15-minute strength-training routine helps build strength and balance in all the major muscle groups in your body. If you're pressed for time, you can split up the routine. Do interval training 1 day, strength training another. Just be sure to leave at least 1 day of rest between strength-training workouts. Turn to Part III of this book for workout plan details.

#7: Plan and track.

Use the journal pages in Part IV of this book to help you plan meals, log what you ate and when you exercised, and keep track of the other benefits of the plan—like a boost in your energy level, mood, and sleep quality. Just like the journal pages for the 5-Day Jump Start, journal pages for Phase 2 give you room to track before-meal hunger and after-meal satisfaction to help you eat more mindfully—a great antidote to emotional eating. Test panelists who kept a food and exercise log found that tracking their meals and exercise made them feel more accountable to themselves, increasing their motivation to make healthy choices.

#8: Follow Phase 2 for 5 weeks by repeating your favorite meals and menus or creating your own the easy way.

In this chapter, you'll find 2 full weeks of Phase 2 menus plus recipes. Each week's menu includes 2 days of low-carb meals and 5 days of regular-carb meals. After the 2 weeks, stay on the plan by choosing your favorite meals from the first 2 weeks already outlined. On low-carb days, you can also go back and reuse favorite low-carb meals from the 5-Day Jump Start. No time for cooking? Eating out? Want to experiment with new ingredients or see how a favorite cookbook recipe stacks up? Use the guidelines and tools in the appendix to create your own meals, to put meals together in a flash, and to eat out with confidence.

2-DAY DIET PHASE 2: LOW-CARB DAYS

Menus and meals on low-carb days add up to 50 grams of carbohydrates per day, as they did on the 5-Day Jump Start. That works out to roughly 15 grams of carbs per meal, plus 5 grams of carbs for a snack.

In our meal plans for Weeks 1 and 2 of Phase 2, low-carb days are always referred to as Days 1 and 2—not because the first 2 days of the week should be your low-carb days. It's just easier for you to find them this way. Remember: On the 2-Day Diet, *you're* in charge. Choose the days that suit *your* preferences, *your* schedule.

Don't want to cook or follow a recipe? Use the mix-and-match chart on pages 200–201 to put together an easy low-carb meal in a flash. Eating out? Check our suggestions for low-carb dining at the nation's largest casual dining and fast-food restaurant chains in Chapter 9. Want to put together your own meals and recipes? Curious about the carb count of a food you'd like to eat? Just consult our reference guide in the appendix to find the carb count (as well as fiber, fat, protein, and calories) in hundreds of everyday foods. We've even provided the "net carbs" in fruits, vegetables, dried beans, and whole grains by subtracting the fiber grams from the total carbohydrate grams. On the 2-Day Diet, use net carbs when determining carb counts.

The 2-Day Diet low-carb menus have their foundation in lean protein, good fats, *and* a surprising variety of fruits, veggies, grains, and dairy products. All low-carb diets depend on protein and fats. These foods have virtually no carbohydrates and deliver nutrients and long-term stomach satisfaction. We've chosen lean sources of protein as well as healthy fats so that these cornerstones work for good health as well as for weight loss. In addition to beef and pork, you'll find skinless poultry and fish on the plan, as well as cheese, which is packed with calcium and vitamin D. And you'll find plenty of low-carb vegetables, including salad greens and leafy greens such as spinach.

The 2-Day Diet difference: Our low-carb menus are specially designed to fit in low-carb, whole grain bread as well as fruit and dairy—in addition to a wide variety of veggies that go beyond the greens, such as tomatoes, mushrooms, and zucchini.

The result? Big flavor. Variety. And the nutrients your body needs. On some other low-carb plans, dairy, grains, and fruit are hard to come by, leading to cravings and unbalanced nutrition. Not here. You'll enjoy toast at breakfast, fruit such as melon and berries, pancakes, even a Strawberry Cream Frostie! And you'll discover just how delicious creative low-carb eating can be—we're talking pizza, steak, Italian meat loaf, stuffed chicken breast, Chinese chicken salad, beef with guacamole, and more.

You'll reap the benefits of low-carb eating without the downsides of full-time low-carb plans that are heavy on meat and fats.

2-DAY DIET PHASE 2: REGULAR-CARB DAYS

On regular-carb days, you'll enjoy *healthy* portions of foods that are packed with natural fiber, good fats, lean protein, and other nutrients proven to assist with weight loss and give you a bodywide health boost. And the foods you get to eat on these days taste great. How about Toasted Cheese and Veggie Pita, Pork Chops with Fresh Sauerkraut, chili-lime shrimp, sweet potato soup, and pasta with mozzarella and peppers? Yum!

Here's an overview of what you'll be eating:

Fruits and vegetables: You'll enjoy more fruits and a wider range of vegetables—including starchy types like potatoes—on regular-carb days. These veggies deliver fiber and a broad range of vitamins, minerals, and antioxidant nutrients proven to prevent disease, fill you up, and help with weight loss and weight maintenance.

Whole grains: You'll also enjoy more whole grains on regular-carb days. This balanced approach means you get the unique range of fiber that whole grains supply—including insoluble fiber for better digestion and after-meal satisfaction, soluble fiber for lowering cholesterol and smoothing the rise in blood sugar after you eat, and specialty fibers like beta-glucan (found in barley, for example) that have a unique, proven ability to keep blood sugar low and steady for hours and help you stay mentally focused. The fiber in whole grains and in produce also helps support your body's natural probiotics—the "good bugs" in your digestive system that keep digestion moving and that emerging research says play important roles in a strong immune system, prevention of depression, and even the maintenance of a healthy weight.[1, 2, 3]

Lean protein: You'll eat slightly smaller portions of lean protein on

Regular-Carb Eating at a Glance

FRUIT:
Eat 2 to 3 servings a day.

1 serving = 1 medium piece of fresh fruit; ½ cup cut, chopped, canned, or frozen fruit; ¼ cup dried fruit; ½ cup 100 percent fruit juice without added sweeteners. Tip: Choose canned and frozen fruits without added sugar.

VEGETABLES:
Eat 4 to 6 servings a day.

1 serving = ½ cup cooked vegetables; 1 cup raw vegetables; ½ cup vegetable juice. Tip: Choose plain frozen vegetables (without butter, cheese, or creamy sauces). Choose reduced-sodium vegetable juice.

WHOLE GRAINS, STARCHY VEGETABLES, AND BEANS:
Eat 3 to 7 servings a day.

1 serving = 1 slice whole grain bread; ½ minibagel, pita, or English muffin; 1 small tortilla; 1 cup whole grain breakfast cereal; 1 medium-size pancake; 1 ounce whole grain crackers; 3 cups air-popped popcorn; ½ cup cooked oatmeal, brown rice, quinoa, barley, whole grain pasta, or hot whole grain cereal; ½ cup cooked corn or lima beans; 1 small potato.

DAIRY:
Eat 2 servings a day.

1 serving = 1 cup low-fat or fat-free milk, calcium-fortified soy or rice milk, or yogurt; 1 ounce cheese; ⅓ cup shredded cheese; ½ cup ricotta or cottage cheese. Tip: Choose low-fat or fat-free dairy products when possible. (Regular-fat dairy products are okay on low-carb days because overall calorie intake is low on those days.)

HEALTHY FATS:
Eat 2 to 3 servings a day.

1 serving = 1 tablespoon olive, canola, or flaxseed oil; 1 tablespoon nut butter; ⅓ cup cubed avocado; 10 olives; 2 ounces dark chocolate; 1 ounce nuts (equals 24 almonds, 18 cashews, 28 peanuts, 20 pecan halves, 46 pistachios, 12 macadamias, or 7 walnut halves). There are also good fats in fatty fish such as salmon, herring, mackerel, sardines, and trout. Tip: In general, limit saturated fats, found in butter. Small amounts of butter are okay on low-carb days.

LEAN/HEALTHY PROTEIN:
Eat 2 to 3 servings a day.

1 serving = 3 ounces beef, reduced-sodium deli meat, lean ground beef, pork, skinless chicken or turkey, fish, or seafood; 1 egg; ¼ cup egg substitute; 3 ounces tofu, tempeh, or other soy food; ½ cup dried beans (legumes such as white, red, black, kidney, and navy beans). Tip: Have a nonmeat protein for one or two meals a day.

regular-carb days, which will make room for more whole grains, produce, and dairy products. But you'll still see lean beef and pork, skinless chicken and turkey, fish and seafood, dried legumes (such as black, red, and white beans), as well as soy products like tofu and tempeh on the menu. These, plus dairy products like low-fat and fat-free yogurt, milk, and cheese, will keep you feeling full and satisfied. And they'll deliver important health-promoting nutrients, such as fiber from beans, calcium and vitamin D from dairy, good fats from some types of fish, B vitamins, and iron from meat and poultry.

Good fats: You'll continue to enjoy good fats on regular-carb days, just as you did on low-carb days. Olive oil, canola oil, nuts, nut butters, and avocado are rich sources of monounsaturated fat that help knock back abdominal fat, control blood sugar, and even rebalance your cholesterol levels (promoting "good" HDLs while controlling "bad" LDLs). You'll get even more good fats when you choose salmon and other fish rich in heart-healthy, brain-smart omega-3 fatty acids.

Low-fat and fat-free dairy products: You'll enjoy more dairy products on regular-carb days than you did on low-carb days. Why? Dairy contains a natural milk sugar called galactose that raises the carb count of your meals. We kept some dairy on low-carb days because bone-building calcium and the all-around health benefits of the vitamin D in dairy are too good to miss. We bumped up the dairy on regular-carb days so you get even more of these benefits. If you don't drink or eat dairy products, you can substitute calcium-enriched soy milk and soy products or choose other calcium-rich plant foods, as outlined in Chapter 5.

Pasta, chocolate, and frozen yogurt: You'll find treats like these scattered throughout the meals and snacks on regular-carb days. Why? This isn't a diet. It's a road map for a lifetime of healthy eating. That means working in foods that would otherwise be considered diet cheats. These foods aren't cheats when you enjoy them in reasonable portions, in the context of a healthy diet. So go ahead and savor real noodles in the Penne Pasta with Roast Peppers and Mozzarella. Bite into a square of dark chocolate or a snack paired with almonds, pecans, or walnuts. Enjoy a cool scoop of frozen yogurt in your favorite flavor, topped with dried fruit and real nuts. Delicious!

What about calories? Regular-carb meal plans deliver 1,500 to 1,800 calories per day. If you prefer to count calories or need to figure out whether a restaurant meal or prepackaged meal from the grocery store will fit in, aim for 450 to 550 calories per meal. Be sure your meal contains healthy ingredients, as outlined in "Regular-Carb Eating at a Glance" on page 121. Same goes for snacks, which can range from 150 to 250 calories.

Stretching Your Wardrobe While You Lose Weight

It's the fashion dilemma you've been waiting for: how to dress yourself (without spending a fortune) while you're in the process of shedding pounds and inches. We've got some clever solutions for every stage.

#1: Bye-bye big stuff. First, your largest-size clothing becomes too baggy. At this stage, turn to formerly snug pieces. Our test panelists rediscovered old favorites at the back of their closets. You'll love slipping into smaller-sized items with ease.

#2: My "snug clothes" are hanging on me! You love the moment your skinny jeans become your new "baggy" jeans. But you still have to get dressed for work, play, and social events. Get busy with needle and thread or your sewing machine (or enlist a talented relative, friend, or local seamstress or tailor) to take tucks along the waists of your favorite pants and skirts. Make creative use of belts and sashes—tuck in your shirt (at last!) and belt your pants or skirt. You can also use waist-defining belts and scarves to quickly nip in a dress that's too big in the middle or to turn a baggy sweater into a form-fitting fashion statement. Turn too-big shirts into over blouses—wear a flattering sweater or cotton T underneath and top with your big shirt.

#3: Help! Nothing fits my new body . . . but I'm not ready to buy a new wardrobe! But you *are* ready to show off your slim physique, even though you're still losing weight. Now's the time to get creative. These budget-friendly steps can bridge the gap:

BORROW, TRADE, OR BARTER. If you have a friend who's around the same size, ask to borrow clothes she doesn't wear regularly. A friend who's losing weight may be interested in trading sizes for a while. Someone with a wardrobe in a size they no longer need may be willing to barter (you get her size 12's, she gets help with her garden, for example.)

SHOP LOCAL CONSIGNMENT AND THRIFT STORES. You can find great-looking clothing at great prices—including new and gently used items. Clothing at consignment shops is often a bit more expensive than thrift-shop finds but may be of higher quality and more recent "vintage." Thrift shops can be a great source for bargain-priced jeans, shorts, shirts, and coats.

ASK ABOUT ALTERATIONS. If you have a closet full of baggy business clothing, research the cost of alterations. Take suits, blazers, and dress pants back to the store where you purchased them—or to a dry cleaner that does alterations—and ask what it would cost to bring them down to your new size. This may be a more affordable way to make these important wardrobe investments last longer.

BUY NEW CLOTHING STRATEGICALLY. Treat yourself to a few useful new essentials—black pants or a few dress shirts for work, a new skirt to wear with a variety of tops. Choose neutral colors in fabrics that bridge the seasons.

Week 1

PANTRY

- Baking powder
- Baking soda
- Canola oil
- Curry powder
- Flaxseeds, ground, or white chia seeds
- Flour, unbleached
- Flour, whole wheat
- Ketchup, reduced-sugar
- Mayonnaise
- Olive oil
- Oregano
- Paprika, smoked
- Pepper
- Rosemary
- Sage
- Salt
- Sesame oil, dark
- Soy sauce, reduced-sodium
- Vinegar, balsamic
- Vinegar, white wine
- Wheat germ, toasted

DAIRY/REFRIGERATED

- Cheese spread, light herbed, 4 ounces
- Cheese, mozzarella, fresh, 2 ounces
- Cheese, Parmesan, grated, 2 ounces
- Cheese, Swiss, reduced-sodium, 2 ounces
- Eggs, large, ½ dozen
- Half-and-half, ½ pint
- Horseradish, prepared
- Milk, low-fat (1%), ½ gallon
- Shirataki noodles, 1 package (8 ounces)
- Yogurt, low-fat (2%), plain, 2 cups
- Yogurt, Greek, low-fat (2%), plain, 1 cup

MEAT, POULTRY, SEAFOOD

- Beef, boneless top round or sirloin, 1 pound
- Chicken breast, boneless, skinless, 1 pound
- Chicken tenders, 1 pound
- Ham steak, reduced-sodium, 8 ounces
- Pork, ground, 1 pound
- Salmon fillets, 4 (6 ounces each)
- Turkey, lean ground, 1 pound
- Turkey sausage, Italian, 8 ounces (loose)

FRUIT

- Apple, 4
- Banana, 5
- Cantaloupe, 1
- Kiwifruit, 1
- Lemon, 3
- Lime, 1
- Mango, 1
- Oranges, 4 (or 3 oranges and 1 cup pineapple chunks)
- Strawberries, 1 pint

VEGETABLES

- Bell pepper, red, 1
- Broccoli rabe, 1 bunch
- Cabbage, green, small head, 1
- Carrots, baby, 1 cup
- Cilantro, 1 bunch
- Cucumber, 2
- Garlic, 1 head
- Ginger, fresh, 3" piece
- Green beans, 1 cup
- Lettuce, romaine, 2 bunches
- Onion, 4
- Parsley, 1 bunch
- Potatoes, new red or Yukon gold, 1½ pounds
- Salad greens, mixed, 2 cups
- Scallions, 2 bunches
- Snow peas, ½ cup
- Tomatoes, plum, 4
- Zucchini, 1

BREAD AND BAKED GOODS

- Bran muffin, 1
- Bread, sliced, low-carb or high-fiber, 1 loaf
- Pita, whole grain (6½"), 1 package
- Wrap, wheat, low-carb or high-fiber, 1 package

FROZEN

- Edamame, shelled, 12 ounces, fresh or frozen
- Yogurt, 1 pint

GROCERIES

- Almond butter, 1 jar
- Almonds, sliced natural, small package
- Anchovies, 1 can (13 ounces)
- Artichoke hearts, marinated, 6 ounces
- Chickpeas, no-salt-added, 1 can (15–19 ounces)
- Low-fat, reduced-sodium chicken or vegetable broth, 1 can (14.5 ounces)
- Oats, quick-cooking, 1 container (18 ounces)
- Rice, wild or wild mix, 1 pound
- Rice cakes, plain, unsalted or lightly salted, 1 bag
- Sesame seeds, small jar or package
- Stewed tomatoes, no-salt-added, 1 can (14.5 ounces)
- Tomato soup, reduced-sodium, 1 can (10¾ ounces)
- Walnuts, chopped, small package

Low-Carb Day

day

1

Check what you ate or write in substitutions below.
(Asterisk indicates recipe provided later in chapter)

BREAKFAST *10 GRAMS CARBOHYDRATES*

	SUBSTITUTIONS/NOTES:
☐ Pork and Apple Sausage*	

Per serving: 372 calories, 20 g protein, 10 g carbohydrates, 28 g fat, 10 g saturated fat, 2 g fiber,
358 mg sodium

RATE YOUR HUNGER BEFORE EATING:	1	2	3	4	5	6	7	8	9	10
RATE YOUR SATISFACTION AFTERWARD:	1	2	3	4	5	6	7	8	9	10

LUNCH *12 GRAMS CARBOHYDRATES*

	SUBSTITUTIONS/NOTES:
☐ 2 ounces sliced fresh mozzarella cheese with	
☐ 1 plum tomato, thinly sliced, and	
☐ 1½ tablespoons Rosemary Balsamic Vinaigrette (page 107)	
☐ 1½ cups mixed greens	
☐ ½ slice low-carb bread	

Per serving: 315 calories, 16 g protein, 12 g carbohydrates, 21 g fat, 6 g saturated fat, 4 g fiber,
142 mg sodium

RATE YOUR HUNGER BEFORE EATING:	1	2	3	4	5	6	7	8	9	10
RATE YOUR SATISFACTION AFTERWARD:	1	2	3	4	5	6	7	8	9	10

DINNER *12 GRAMS CARBOHYDRATES*

	SUBSTITUTIONS/NOTES:

☐ Beef and Scallion Stir-Fry*
☐ ½ cup shirataki noodles

Per serving: 389 calories, 38 g protein, 12 g carbohydrates, 20 g fat, 6 g saturated fat, 5 g fiber, 416 mg sodium

RATE YOUR HUNGER BEFORE EATING:	1 2 3 4 5 6 7 8 9 10
RATE YOUR SATISFACTION AFTERWARD:	1 2 3 4 5 6 7 8 9 10

SNACK *15 GRAMS CARBOHYDRATES*

	SUBSTITUTIONS/NOTES:

☐ 1 Strawberry Cream Frostie*

Per serving: 148 calories, 4 g protein, 15 g carbohydrates, 9 g fat, 4 g saturated fat, 5 g fiber, 26 mg sodium

RATE YOUR HUNGER BEFORE EATING:	1 2 3 4 5 6 7 8 9 10
RATE YOUR SATISFACTION AFTERWARD:	1 2 3 4 5 6 7 8 9 10

Per day: 1,224 calories, 78 g protein, 50 g carbohydrates, 81 g fat, 29 g saturated fat, 17 g fiber, 951 mg sodium, 328 mg calcium, 4 IU vitamin D

day
2

Low-Carb Day

Check what you ate or write in substitutions below.
(Asterisk indicates recipe provided later in chapter)

BREAKFAST *17 GRAMS CARBOHYDRATES*

	SUBSTITUTIONS/NOTES:
☐ 2 soft-cooked eggs ☐ 1 slice low-carb toast with ☐ 1 teaspoon butter ☐ 6 ounces low-fat milk or yogurt	

Per serving: 321 calories, 22 g protein, 17 g carbohydrates, 19 g fat, 7 g saturated fat, 3 g fiber,
401 mg sodium

RATE YOUR HUNGER BEFORE EATING:	1 2 3 4 5 6 7 8 9 10
RATE YOUR SATISFACTION AFTERWARD:	1 2 3 4 5 6 7 8 9 10

LUNCH *17 GRAMS CARBOHYDRATES*

	SUBSTITUTIONS/NOTES:
☐ 1 serving Chinese Chicken Salad* ☐ 2 cups mixed greens ☐ ½ cup orange sections	

Per serving: 396 calories, 40 g protein, 17 g carbohydrates, 19 g fat, 3 g saturated fat, 6 g fiber,
116 mg sodium

RATE YOUR HUNGER BEFORE EATING:	1 2 3 4 5 6 7 8 9 10
RATE YOUR SATISFACTION AFTERWARD:	1 2 3 4 5 6 7 8 9 10

DINNER *12 GRAMS CARBOHYDRATES*

	SUBSTITUTIONS/NOTES:
☐ Italian Sausage Meat Loaf*	
☐ 1 carrot cut in chunks and roasted in	
☐ 2 teaspoons olive oil	

Per serving: 365 calories, 41 g protein, 12 g carbohydrates, 19 g fat, 2 g saturated fat, 2 g fiber,
663 mg sodium

RATE YOUR HUNGER BEFORE EATING: 1   2   3   4   5   6   7   8   9   10
RATE YOUR SATISFACTION AFTERWARD: 1   2   3   4   5   6   7   8   9   10

SNACK *4 GRAMS CARBOHYDRATES*

	SUBSTITUTIONS/NOTES:
☐ 1 cup cucumber round with	
☐ 1½ tablespoons light herbed cheese spread	

Per serving: 59 calories, 2 g protein, 4 g carbohydrates, 4 g fat, 2 g saturated fat, 1 g fiber,
122 mg sodium

RATE YOUR HUNGER BEFORE EATING: 1   2   3   4   5   6   7   8   9   10
RATE YOUR SATISFACTION AFTERWARD: 1   2   3   4   5   6   7   8   9   10

Per day: 1,142 calories, 105 g protein, 50 g carbohydrates, 60 g fat, 14 g saturated fat, 13 g fiber,
1,303 mg sodium, 636 mg calcium, 68 IU vitamin D

Regular-Carb Day

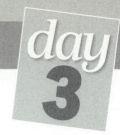

day
3

Check what you ate or write in substitutions below.
(Asterisk indicates recipe provided later in chapter)

BREAKFAST

	SUBSTITUTIONS/NOTES:
☐ Creamy, Cheesy Scrambled Eggs* ☐ 1 medium orange	

Per serving: 372 calories, 20 g protein, 23 g carbohydrates, 23 g fat, 8 g saturated fat, 3 g fiber,
832 mg sodium

RATE YOUR HUNGER BEFORE EATING:	1	2	3	4	5	6	7	8	9	10
RATE YOUR SATISFACTION AFTERWARD:	1	2	3	4	5	6	7	8	9	10

LUNCH

	SUBSTITUTIONS/NOTES:
☐ 1 cup salad bar pasta salad with cherry tomatoes and broccoli ☐ 3 ounces cooked chicken or turkey ☐ 2-3 cups mixed salad greens ☐ 1 tablespoon Caesar Dressing* ☐ 1 apple or pear	

Per serving: 521 calories, 35 g protein, 56 g carbohydrates, 19 g fat, 3 g saturated fat, 9 g fiber,
467 mg sodium

RATE YOUR HUNGER BEFORE EATING:	1	2	3	4	5	6	7	8	9	10
RATE YOUR SATISFACTION AFTERWARD:	1	2	3	4	5	6	7	8	9	10

DINNER

	SUBSTITUTIONS/NOTES:
☐ Curried Chickpeas and Potatoes*	
☐ 2 cups mixed greens with cucumber and radishes	
☐ Lime Vinaigrette (page 111)	

Per serving: 467 calories, 10 g protein, 36 g carbohydrates, 32 g fat, 5 g saturated fat, 9 g fiber, 696 mg sodium

RATE YOUR HUNGER BEFORE EATING:	1 2 3 4 5 6 7 8 9 10
RATE YOUR SATISFACTION AFTERWARD:	1 2 3 4 5 6 7 8 9 10

SNACK

	SUBSTITUTIONS/NOTES:
☐ 2 rice cakes with	
☐ 2 tablespoons almond butter	

Per serving: 268 calories, 6 g protein, 22 g carbohydrates, 19 g fat, 2 g saturated fat, 2 g fiber, 168 mg sodium

RATE YOUR HUNGER BEFORE EATING:	1 2 3 4 5 6 7 8 9 10
RATE YOUR SATISFACTION AFTERWARD:	1 2 3 4 5 6 7 8 9 10

Per day: 1,628 calories, 71 g protein, 137 g carbohydrates, 93 g fat, 17 g saturated fat, 23 g fiber, 2,164 mg sodium, 578 mg calcium, 59 IU vitamin D

day 4

Regular-Carb Day

Check what you ate or write in substitutions below.
(Asterisk indicates recipe provided later in chapter)

BREAKFAST

	SUBSTITUTIONS/NOTES:
☐ 1 cup oatmeal	
☐ 1 cup strawberries (about 6 large), cut in half	
☐ 1 cup 1% low-fat milk	

Per serving: 317 calories, 15 g protein, 52 g carbohydrates, 6 g fat, 2 g saturated fat, 7 g fiber, 275 mg sodium

RATE YOUR HUNGER BEFORE EATING:	1 2 3 4 5 6 7 8 9 10
RATE YOUR SATISFACTION AFTERWARD:	1 2 3 4 5 6 7 8 9 10

LUNCH

	SUBSTITUTIONS/NOTES:
☐ 1 cup tomato soup	
☐ Wild Rice Salad with Ham and Apple*	

Per serving: 523 calories, 22 g protein, 58 g carbohydrates, 25 g fat, 5 g saturated fat, 7 g fiber, 1,234 mg sodium

RATE YOUR HUNGER BEFORE EATING:	1 2 3 4 5 6 7 8 9 10
RATE YOUR SATISFACTION AFTERWARD:	1 2 3 4 5 6 7 8 9 10

DINNER

	SUBSTITUTIONS/NOTES:
☐ Grilled Salmon with Cucumber-Horseradish Sauce*	
☐ ½ cup steamed new red or Yukon gold potatoes	
☐ 1 cup steamed green beans	

Per serving: 429 calories, 40 g protein, 30 g carbohydrates, 16 g fat, 3 g saturated fat, 5 g fiber, 298 mg sodium

RATE YOUR HUNGER BEFORE EATING:	1	2	3	4	5	6	7	8	9	10
RATE YOUR SATISFACTION AFTERWARD:	1	2	3	4	5	6	7	8	9	10

SNACK

	SUBSTITUTIONS/NOTES:
☐ 1 ounce dark chocolate (at least 60% cocoa)	
☐ 15 walnuts or almonds	

Per serving: 347 calories, 6 g protein, 19 g carbohydrates, 31 g fat, 8 g saturated fat, 4 g fiber, 1 mg sodium

RATE YOUR HUNGER BEFORE EATING:	1	2	3	4	5	6	7	8	9	10
RATE YOUR SATISFACTION AFTERWARD:	1	2	3	4	5	6	7	8	9	10

Per day: 1,616 calories, 83 g protein, 159 g carbohydrates, 78 g fat, 19 g saturated fat, 23 g fiber, 1,807 mg sodium, 624 mg calcium, 21 IU vitamin D

Regular-Carb Day

Check what you ate or write in substitutions below.
(Asterisk indicates recipe provided later in chapter)

BREAKFAST

☐ 1 Orange–Wheat Germ Biscuit*
spread with

☐ 1 teaspoon butter

☐ 1 cup low-fat plain yogurt blended
with

☐ 1 cup blueberries or raspberries

SUBSTITUTIONS/NOTES:

Per serving: 502 calories, 21 g protein, 64 g carbohydrates, 20 g fat, 7 g saturated fat, 8 g fiber,
684 mg sodium

RATE YOUR HUNGER BEFORE EATING:	1	2	3	4	5	6	7	8	9	10
RATE YOUR SATISFACTION AFTERWARD:	1	2	3	4	5	6	7	8	9	10

LUNCH

☐ 1 slice pizza

☐ 1 cup tossed green salad with

☐ 1 tablespoon light dressing

☐ 1 orange or 1 cup pineapple chunks

SUBSTITUTIONS/NOTES:

Per serving: 421 calories, 17 g protein, 49 g carbohydrates, 18 g fat, 7 g saturated fat, 5 g fiber,
941 mg sodium

RATE YOUR HUNGER BEFORE EATING:	1	2	3	4	5	6	7	8	9	10
RATE YOUR SATISFACTION AFTERWARD:	1	2	3	4	5	6	7	8	9	10

DINNER

	SUBSTITUTIONS/NOTES:
☐ Lemon-Herb Chicken Tenders*	
☐ 1 cup brown rice	
☐ 1 cup sautéed zucchini and cherry tomatoes in 2 teaspoons olive oil	

Per serving: 492 calories, 33 g protein, 52 g carbohydrates, 19 g fat, 3 g saturated fat, 6 g fiber, 210 mg sodium

RATE YOUR HUNGER BEFORE EATING: 1 2 3 4 5 6 7 8 9 10
RATE YOUR SATISFACTION AFTERWARD: 1 2 3 4 5 6 7 8 9 10

SNACK

	SUBSTITUTIONS/NOTES:
☐ ½ cup Roasted Edamame*	

Per serving: 117 calories, 9 g protein, 8 g carbohydrates, 6 g fat, 0 g saturated fat, 4 g fiber, 151 mg sodium

RATE YOUR HUNGER BEFORE EATING: 1 2 3 4 5 6 7 8 9 10
RATE YOUR SATISFACTION AFTERWARD: 1 2 3 4 5 6 7 8 9 10

Per day: 1,532 calories, 80 g protein, 174 g carbohydrates, 63 g fat, 17 g saturated fat, 24 g fiber, 1,985 mg sodium, 946 mg calcium, 5 IU vitamin D

Regular-Carb Day

Check what you ate or write in substitutions below.
(Asterisk indicates recipe provided later in chapter)

BREAKFAST

	SUBSTITUTIONS/NOTES:
☐ 1 banana, split and spread with	
☐ 1 tablespoon almond butter	
☐ 1 kiwi	
☐ 1 cup 1% low-fat milk or yogurt	

Per serving: 349 calories, 13 g protein, 53 g carbohydrates, 12 g fat, 3 g saturated fat, 6 g fiber,
181 mg sodium

RATE YOUR HUNGER BEFORE EATING:	1 2 3 4 5 6 7 8 9 10
RATE YOUR SATISFACTION AFTERWARD:	1 2 3 4 5 6 7 8 9 10

LUNCH

	SUBSTITUTIONS/NOTES:
☐ Chef Salad Wrap*	
☐ ½ cup sliced apple	

Per serving: 418 calories, 33 g protein, 33 g carbohydrates, 24 g fat, 8 g saturated fat, 15 g fiber,
486 mg sodium

RATE YOUR HUNGER BEFORE EATING:	1 2 3 4 5 6 7 8 9 10
RATE YOUR SATISFACTION AFTERWARD:	1 2 3 4 5 6 7 8 9 10

DINNER

	SUBSTITUTIONS/NOTES:
☐ 2 cups romaine lettuce salad with	
☐ Greek Vinaigrette (page 105)*	
☐ Beef and Vegetable Roast*	

Per serving: 828 calories, 52 g protein, 40 g carbohydrates, 51 g fat, 12 g saturated fat, 7 g fiber,
518 mg sodium

RATE YOUR HUNGER BEFORE EATING:	1	2	3	4	5	6	7	8	9	10
RATE YOUR SATISFACTION AFTERWARD:	1	2	3	4	5	6	7	8	9	10

SNACK

	SUBSTITUTIONS/NOTES:
☐ ½ cup vanilla frozen yogurt with	
☐ 1 tablespoon chopped walnuts	

Per serving: 188 calories, 4 g protein, 22 g carbohydrates, 9 g fat, 3 g saturated fat, 0.5 g fiber,
45 mg sodium

RATE YOUR HUNGER BEFORE EATING:	1	2	3	4	5	6	7	8	9	10
RATE YOUR SATISFACTION AFTERWARD:	1	2	3	4	5	6	7	8	9	10

Per day: 1,783 calories, 102 g protein, 147 g carbohydrates, 96 g fat, 26 g saturated fat, 29 g fiber,
1,229 mg sodium, 1,004 mg calcium, 36 IU vitamin D

day 7

Regular-Carb Day

Check what you ate or write in substitutions below.
(Asterisk indicates recipe provided later in chapter)

BREAKFAST

	SUBSTITUTIONS/NOTES:
☐ Roast Beef Hash* ☐ 1 medium orange	

Per serving: 340 calories, 23 g protein, 35 g carbohydrates, 12 g fat, 3 g saturated fat, 5 g fiber,
328 mg sodium

RATE YOUR HUNGER BEFORE EATING:	1 2 3 4 5 6 7 8 9 10
RATE YOUR SATISFACTION AFTERWARD:	1 2 3 4 5 6 7 8 9 10

LUNCH

	SUBSTITUTIONS/NOTES:
☐ Toasted Cheese and Veggie Pita* ☐ 1 medium apple	

Per serving: 480 calories, 29 g protein, 49 g carbohydrates, 21 g fat, 10 g saturated fat, 15 g fiber,
699 mg sodium

RATE YOUR HUNGER BEFORE EATING:	1 2 3 4 5 6 7 8 9 10
RATE YOUR SATISFACTION AFTERWARD:	1 2 3 4 5 6 7 8 9 10

DINNER

SUBSTITUTIONS/NOTES:

☐ Pork Chops with Fresh Sauerkraut*
☐ 1 cup mashed potato
☐ 1 cup steamed asparagus or spinach

Per serving: 524 calories, 32 g protein, 54 g carbohydrates, 21 g fat, 7 g saturated fat, 9 g fiber,
1,012 mg sodium

RATE YOUR HUNGER BEFORE EATING: 1 2 3 4 5 6 7 8 9 10
RATE YOUR SATISFACTION AFTERWARD: 1 2 3 4 5 6 7 8 9 10

SNACK

SUBSTITUTIONS/NOTES:

☐ 1 cup 2% plain Greek yogurt blended
   with
☐ ½ tablespoon cocoa powder and
☐ 2 teaspoons sugar

Per serving: 168 calories, 18 g protein, 18 g carbohydrates, 4 g fat, 3 g saturated fat, 1 g fiber,
66 mg sodium

RATE YOUR HUNGER BEFORE EATING: 1 2 3 4 5 6 7 8 9 10
RATE YOUR SATISFACTION AFTERWARD: 1 2 3 4 5 6 7 8 9 10

Per day: 1,513 calories, 102 g protein, 156 g carbohydrates, 58 g fat, 24 g saturated fat, 31 g fiber,
2,105 mg sodium, 945 mg calcium, 89 IU vitamin D

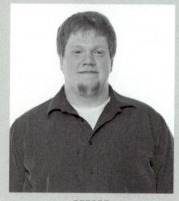

BEFORE

"This Has Been a Big Awakening!"

Matt Opatovsky had some bad news for his mother. Just before his 24th birthday, he called to ask her not to bake him a birthday cake this year . . . but how about whipping up some hummus instead? "My mom's a former baker, so it was kind of devastating when I told her I was eating low-carb for a couple of weeks and didn't want a cake this time," he says. "It was a big deal. She did make me two big containers of hummus, with fresh garlic and lots of tahini, just the way I like it." And she even put a candle on top!

That very nontraditional birthday treat helped Matt reach a 20.8-pound weight loss. "Eating this way has been a big awakening for me," he says. "I'm reading nutrition labels now, and I'm making choices based on the number of carbs and the amount of sugar in foods. It's changed the way I eat."

Matt started keeping string cheese, baby carrots, and nuts on hand for snacks when he got hungry at work. And he gave up the 32-ounce sweetened iced coffee drinks he used to stop for every morning on the way to his job as a sales analyst. "I don't drink much soda—maybe on a special occasion—and I didn't drink diet soda, either," he says. "But I used to drink a lot of big coffee drinks and a lot of prepared, sweetened iced tea, which I now realize is as sweet as soda. Now I go for unsweetened tea and have more water. It feels good."

Despite his impressive weight loss, Matt says the

experience of the program was even more important to him. "I've learned a lot about food," he notes. And he found ways to adapt the recipes, too. "I used the meal plans as an inspiration," he says. "As a single guy, I didn't want to make a four-serving entrée. So I made meals based on the plan."

Breakfast was often eggs cooked with onions and peppers. Lunch was no longer fast food or a big sandwich. Instead, he might have a salad and some meat. Dinner? Lean protein and veggies—like grilled or baked chicken with carrots, asparagus, celery, and hummus.

"I really like ethnic cuisine, but I'll make it myself in a healthy way now instead of getting Chinese or Indian take-out," he says. He also gave away his bread and pasta at the start of the program. Now, he'll have low-carb shirataki noodles or spaghetti squash with his pasta sauce and make the occasional sandwich with a high-fiber wrap. "It's about making better choices," he says. "I don't bring home food from the grocery store that isn't healthy. I don't want to tempt myself."

His advice: "Don't get discouraged if you can't stick to the plan exactly. And don't get thrown off if you have an off day. Just recover and get back on it. It'll work."

Pork and Apple Sausage

Delicious on low-carb days, this family favorite works any day of the week but is especially good on weekend mornings, when you may have more time to enjoy cooking breakfast.

PREP TIME: 15 MINUTES ■ TOTAL TIME: 20 MINUTES

1 large apple, peeled and shredded

1 small onion, finely chopped

1 pound ground pork

1½ teaspoons dried sage

½ teaspoon salt

1 tablespoon olive oil

1. Place the apple and onion in a large bowl.

2. Add the pork, sage, and salt and combine. Shape into 8 patties.

3. Heat the oil in a large skillet over medium-high heat. Add the patties and cook, turning once, for 5 to 6 minutes, or until no longer pink.

MAKES 4 SERVINGS (2 PATTIES EACH)

PER SERVING: 372 calories, 20 g protein, 10 g carbohydrates, 28 g fat, 10 g saturated fat, 2 g fiber, 358 mg sodium

Creamy, Cheesy Scrambled Eggs

A breakfast standard gets a fancy, satisfying upgrade with scallions and two kinds of cheese.

PREP TIME: 5 MINUTES ■ TOTAL TIME: 10 MINUTES

4 eggs

2 tablespoons low-fat milk

¼ cup ricotta cheese

2 tablespoons grated Parmesan cheese

2 scallions, thinly sliced

½ teaspoon salt

1 tablespoon olive oil

1. In a large bowl, beat the eggs and milk. Add the cheeses, scallions, and salt and mix well.

2. Heat the oil in a large skillet over medium heat. Add the egg mixture and cook, stirring with a fork to scramble, for 3 to 5 minutes, or until the eggs are set.

MAKES 2 SERVINGS

PER SERVING: 292 calories, 19 g protein, 4 g carbohydrates, 23 g fat, 8 g saturated fat, 0 g fiber, 832 mg sodium

Orange–Wheat Germ Biscuits

Wake up to delicately scented biscuits—delicious with coffee or tea. You can substitute dried, grated orange peel; follow the label directions for the right amount to replace freshly grated peel.

PREP TIME: 15 MINUTES ■ TOTAL TIME: 25 MINUTES

¼ cup + 1 tablespoon olive oil

1½ cups whole grain pastry flour

½ cup toasted wheat germ

2 tablespoons ground golden flaxseed

1 tablespoon baking powder

½ teaspoon salt

½ cup low-fat plain yogurt

2 teaspoons freshly grated orange peel

1. Preheat the oven to 450°F. Lightly grease a baking sheet with 1 tablespoon of the oil (you may need less).

2. In a large bowl, combine the flour, wheat germ, flaxseed, baking powder, and salt.

3. Stir in the yogurt, orange peel, and the remaining ¼ cup oil.

4. Lightly flour a cutting board. Pat the biscuit dough into a square on the cutting board, then cut evenly into 6 biscuits. Place on the baking sheet and bake for 10 to 12 minutes, or until lightly browned.

MAKES 6 SERVINGS

PER SERVING: 230 calories, 7 g protein, 26 g carbohydrates, 12 g fat, 1.5 g saturated fat, 4 g fiber, 484 mg sodium

Roast Beef Hash

You can make this tasty and economical hash with leftovers from your Beef and Vegetable Roast dinner (page 155), or use cooked leftover turkey, chicken, or fish (use steaks like salmon or tuna) for a change of pace.

PREP TIME: 10 MINUTES ■ TOTAL TIME: 15 MINUTES

1½ cups cooked roast beef, chopped

1½ cups cooked and cubed potatoes, chopped

1 red bell pepper, chopped

1 onion, chopped

½ teaspoon salt

¼ teaspoon ground black pepper

1 tablespoon olive oil

1. In a bowl, combine the beef, potatoes, bell pepper, onion, salt, and black pepper.

2. Heat the oil in a large skillet over medium heat. Add the beef mixture and heat, stirring so it doesn't stick, for 5 minutes, or until heated through.

MAKES 4 SERVINGS

PER SERVING: 260 calories, 22 g protein, 16 g carbohydrates, 12 g fat, 3 g saturated fat, 2 g fiber, 328 mg sodium

Chinese Chicken Salad

Turn leftover chicken into a fast and elegant midday meal.

PREP TIME: 10 MINUTES ■ TOTAL TIME: 10 MINUTES

1 pound (4 cups) cooked and chopped boneless, skinless chicken breast

2 scallions, thickly sliced

¼ cup fresh cilantro, finely chopped

¼ cup sliced natural almonds

2 tablespoons toasted sesame seeds

3 tablespoons olive oil

1½ tablespoons rice wine vinegar

1. In a large bowl, combine the chicken, scallions, cilantro, almonds, and sesame seeds.

2. Drizzle with the oil and vinegar, then toss to mix.

MAKES 4 SERVINGS

PER SERVING: 335 calories, 37 g protein, 3 g carbohydrates, 19 g fat, 3 g saturated fat, 2 g fiber, 88 mg sodium

Toasted Cheese and Veggie Pita

Add fiber and flavor to toasted cheese with artichokes and more.

PREP TIME: 5 MINUTES ■ TOTAL TIME: 10 MINUTES

1 (6½") low-carb or high-fiber pita

½ cup shredded romaine lettuce

2 thin slices tomato

2 drained marinated artichoke hearts

2 ounces reduced-sodium Swiss cheese

1. Slice a thin strip from one edge of the pita, so that you can insert ingredients into the "pocket" in the bread.

2. Stuff with the lettuce, tomato, artichoke hearts, and cheese.

3. Coat a large skillet or nonstick sandwich grill with cooking spray. Cook the pita, turning once, for 5 minutes.

MAKES 1 SERVING

PER SERVING: 386 calories, 29 g protein, 23 g carbohydrates, 20 g fat, 10 g saturated fat, 11 g fiber, 697 mg sodium

Wild Rice Salad with Ham and Apple

The autumn-inspired flavor of this hearty salad is good any time of year.

PREP TIME: 30 MINUTES ▪ TOTAL TIME: 30 MINUTES

Wild rice mix (enough to make 3 cups, cooked)

8 ounces lean, reduced-sodium ham, chopped into small pieces

1 large apple, chopped

½ cup walnuts, chopped

2 tablespoons olive oil

1 tablespoon fresh lemon juice

1. Cook the wild rice mix according to package directions.

2. In a large bowl, combine the rice, ham, apple, and walnuts. Drizzle with the oil and lemon juice, then toss to mix.

MAKES 4 SERVINGS

PER SERVING: 403 calories, 20 g protein, 37 g carbohydrates, 21 g fat, 3.5 g saturated fat, 5 g fiber, 554 mg sodium

Chef Salad Wrap

A hearty deli favorite just got healthier!

PREP TIME: 15 MINUTES ■ TOTAL TIME: 15 MINUTES

1 cup shredded romaine lettuce

½ cup chopped tomato

1 hard-cooked egg, sliced

1 ounce roast chicken breast or lean roast beef

1 ounce reduced-sodium Swiss cheese

1 (10") low-carb or high-fiber wheat wrap

1 tablespoon Greek Vinaigrette (page 105) or Caesar Dressing (recipe follows)

1. Arrange the lettuce, tomato, egg, chicken or beef, and cheese on the wrap.

2. Drizzle with Greek Vinaigrette or Caesar Dressing, roll up, and enjoy.

MAKES 1 SERVING

PER SERVING: 389 calories, 33 g protein, 25 g carbohydrates, 23 g fat, 8 g saturated fat, 14 g fiber, 485 mg sodium

Caesar Dressing

Keep the dressing in a bottle in the refrigerator so it's ready when you need it.

PREP TIME: 5 MINUTES ■ TOTAL TIME: 5 MINUTES

½ cup olive oil

¼ cup olive oil mayonnaise

2 tablespoons white vinegar

4 cloves garlic, sliced

1 anchovy fillet

¼ teaspoon salt

⅛ teaspoon pepper

Combine all of the ingredients in a blender and whirl until smooth. Store in a container with a tight-fitting lid in the refrigerator. Shake before using.

MAKES 12 (1-TABLESPOON) SERVINGS

PER SERVING: 115 calories, 0 g protein, 0 g carbohydrates, 13 g fat, 2 g saturated fat, 0 g fiber, 88 mg sodium

Beef and Scallion Stir-Fry

To save time getting dinner on the table at night, cut up the steak in advance and allow it to marinate in the refrigerator all day.

PREP TIME: 20 MINUTES PLUS MARINATING TIME
■ TOTAL TIME: 25 MINUTES PLUS MARINATING TIME

2 tablespoons reduced-sodium soy sauce

3 cloves garlic, finely chopped

2 tablespoons minced fresh ginger

1½ pounds trimmed boneless top round or sirloin steak, thinly sliced across the grain

2 tablespoons olive oil

1 bunch scallions, cut into 1½" pieces

4 cups shredded green cabbage

1. In a medium bowl, combine the soy sauce, garlic, and ginger. Add the beef and stir to coat. Cover the bowl and marinate for 30 minutes at room temperature or at least 1 hour in the refrigerator.

2. Heat the oil in a wok or large skillet over medium-high heat. With a slotted spoon, transfer the beef to the wok, reserving the marinade. Cook the beef, stirring constantly, for 1 to 2 minutes, or until browned on all sides. Remove the beef to a plate. Set aside and keep warm.

3. Add the scallions to the wok and cook, stirring constantly, for 30 seconds. Add the reserved marinade and cook for 1 minute, stirring constantly to avoid burning. Add the beef and cabbage and cook, stirring constantly, for 2 minutes, or until cooked through.

MAKES 4 SERVINGS

PER SERVING: 263 calories, 37 g protein, 8 g carbohydrates, 20 g fat, 6 g saturated fat, 3 g fiber, 396 mg sodium

Italian Sausage Meat Loaf

Adding sausage and ketchup to a meat loaf mixture provides wonderful flavor. And mushrooms and onions improve the texture just as well as the starchier bread crumbs or oatmeal traditionally used to prevent the loaf from becoming too dense.

PREP TIME: 10 MINUTES ■ TOTAL TIME: 1 HOUR

1 pound lean ground turkey breast

½ pound hot or sweet Italian turkey sausage (loose)

2 cups mushrooms, finely chopped

1 onion, finely chopped

1 egg

¼ cup reduced-sugar ketchup

¼ cup finely chopped fresh basil or parsley, or 1 teaspoon dried

1. Preheat the oven to 350°F. Line a shallow baking pan with aluminum foil. Coat the foil with cooking spray.

2. In a large bowl, combine the turkey breast, sausage, mushrooms, onion, egg, ketchup, and parsley. Shape into a loaf and place in the pan.

3. Bake for 50 minutes, or until a thermometer inserted in the center registers 165°F and the meat is no longer pink.

MAKES 4 SERVINGS

PER SERVING: 260 calories, 40 g protein, 6 g carbohydrates, 9 g fat, 0.5 g saturated fat, 1 g fiber, 621 mg sodium

Curried Chickpeas and Potatoes

If you don't have curry powder, you can substitute 1 teaspoon each of ground cumin and ground coriander.

PREP TIME: 10 MINUTES ■ TOTAL TIME: 35 MINUTES

1 tablespoon olive oil

1 onion, finely chopped

2 teaspoons curry powder

8 ounces new red or Yukon gold potatoes, chopped

1 can (14.5 ounces) low-fat, reduced-sodium chicken or vegetable broth

1 can (14.5 ounces) no-salt-added stewed or diced tomatoes

1 can (15–19 ounces) no-salt-added chickpeas

½ teaspoon salt

¼ cup finely chopped cilantro

1. Heat the oil in a large skillet over medium heat. Add the onion and cook for 5 minutes, or until tender. Add the curry powder and potatoes and cook, stirring, for 1 minute.

2. Add the broth and the tomatoes and simmer, stirring occasionally, for 15 minutes, or until the potatoes are tender.

3. Add the chickpeas and salt and cook, stirring occasionally, for 3 minutes, or until heated through. Stir in the cilantro.

MAKES 4 SERVINGS

PER SERVING: 200 calories, 8 g protein, 31 g carbohydrates, 5 g fat, 1 g saturated fat, 6 g fiber, 371 mg sodium

Grilled Salmon with Cucumber-Horseradish Sauce

Instead of the usual dill sauce for salmon, try this spicy alternative!

PREP TIME: 10 MINUTES ■ TOTAL TIME: 20 MINUTES

Sauce

- ½ cup low-fat plain yogurt
- 2 tablespoons fresh lemon juice
- 2 tablespoons mayonnaise
- 1 tablespoon prepared horseradish
- ¼ teaspoon salt
- ½ cucumber, peeled and finely chopped

Salmon

- 4 (6-ounce) salmon fillets
- 1 tablespoon olive oil

1. *To make the sauce:* In a small bowl, combine the yogurt, lemon juice, mayonnaise, horseradish, and salt. Mix in the cucumber. Set aside.

2. *To make the salmon:* Coat a grill rack or broiler-pan rack with cooking spray. Preheat the grill or broiler. Brush the salmon fillets with the oil. Grill or broil for 6 to 8 minutes, turning once, or until the fish is just opaque.

3. Serve the salmon topped with the sauce, or serve the sauce on the side.

MAKES 4 SERVINGS

PER SERVING: 315 calories, 36 g protein, 5 g carbohydrates, 16 g fat, 3 g saturated fat, 0 g fiber, 291 mg sodium

Lemon-Herb Chicken Tenders

Keep chicken tenders in the freezer for quick weeknight meals. They defrost in a flash in the microwave. Here's how to make them a family favorite.

PREP TIME: 5 MINUTES PLUS MARINATING TIME
TOTAL TIME: 10 MINUTES PLUS MARINATING TIME

¼ cup fresh lemon juice

2 tablespoons olive oil

2 teaspoons dried oregano, crumbled

¼ teaspoon salt

1 pound chicken tenders

1. In a large bowl, combine the lemon juice, oil, oregano, and salt. Add the chicken tenders, cover, and marinate for 30 minutes at room temperature or 1 hour in the refrigerator.

2. Coat a grill rack or broiler-pan rack with cooking spray. Preheat the grill or broiler. Grill or broil the chicken 4" from the heat source, turning once, for 5 minutes, or until no longer pink and the juices run clear.

MAKES 4 SERVINGS

PER SERVING: 170 calories, 26 g protein, 2 g carbohydrates, 7 g fat, 1 g saturated fat, 0 g fiber, 193 mg sodium

Beef and Vegetable Roast

Unless you are feeding eight people, you will have enough leftovers to make Roast Beef Hash for breakfast and Roast Beef and Guacamole in Lettuce Boats for lunch in the upcoming week.

PREP TIME: 20 MINUTES ▪ TOTAL TIME: 1 HOUR 50 MINUTES

4 pounds rib-eye beef roast

3 tablespoons olive oil, divided

4 cloves garlic, finely chopped, divided

1 tablespoon dried rosemary, crumbled, divided

1 teaspoon salt, divided

¼ teaspoon ground black pepper

3 pounds small new red potatoes, halved

1 package (1 pound) baby carrots

1 head cauliflower, trimmed and separated into florets

1. Preheat the oven to 350°F. Coat a large shallow roasting pan with cooking spray.

2. Place the beef in the pan and rub with 1 tablespoon of the oil, half of the garlic, and 1 teaspoon of the rosemary. Sprinkle with ½ teaspoon of the salt and the pepper.

3. In a large bowl, combine the potatoes, carrots, and cauliflower with the remaining 2 tablespoons oil, garlic, 2 teaspoons rosemary, and ½ teaspoon salt. Spread the vegetables in a single layer around the roast.

4. Roast the beef and vegetables for 1 hour to 1 hour and 30 minutes, or until the vegetables are tender and a thermometer inserted in the center of the roast registers 145°F for medium-rare/160°F for medium/165°F for well-done. Let the roast stand for 10 minutes before slicing. Serve with the vegetables.

MAKES 8 SERVINGS

PER SERVING: 571 calories, 51 g protein, 36 g carbohydrates, 24 g fat, 8 g saturated fat, 6 g fiber, 511 mg sodium

Pork Chops with Fresh Sauerkraut

You'll never go back to canned or packaged sauerkraut once you discover how fast and tasty the fresh stuff really is!

PREP TIME: 15 MINUTES ■ TOTAL TIME: 25 MINUTES

1 tablespoon olive oil

4 center-cut boneless loin pork chops (about 1 pound total)

4 cups thinly sliced green cabbage

1 onion, thinly sliced

3 cloves garlic, finely chopped

¼ cup apple cider vinegar

¼ cup water

2 teaspoons caraway seeds

½ teaspoon salt

1. Heat the oil in a large skillet over medium heat. Cook the pork chops for 1 minute on each side, or until lightly browned. Remove the chops from the skillet, set aside, and keep warm.

2. Add the cabbage, onion, and garlic to the skillet and cook for 5 minutes, stirring occasionally, or until just wilted. Stir in the vinegar, water, caraway seeds, and salt. Cook for 1 minute.

3. Return the pork chops to the skillet. Cover and cook for 2 minutes, or until a thermometer inserted in the center of a chop registers 160°F and the juices run clear.

MAKES 4 SERVINGS

PER SERVING: 311 calories, 24 g protein, 10 g carbohydrates, 20 g fat, 6 g saturated fat, 3 g fiber, 353 mg sodium

Pineapple Chicken Stir-Fry

You can substitute snow peas, scallions, or green peppers for the red peppers in this recipe or use a combination of vegetables. This dish is equally delicious made with chunks of pork tenderloin instead of chicken.

PREP TIME: 10 MINUTES ■ TOTAL TIME: 20 MINUTES

2 tablespoons no-salt-added tomato paste

1 tablespoon low-sodium soy sauce

1 tablespoon honey mustard

2 cloves garlic, finely chopped

1 can (1 pound, 4 ounces) pineapple chunks in juice, drained, with juice reserved

1 pound boneless, skinless chicken breast, cut into bite-size pieces

1 tablespoon olive or sesame oil

1 red bell pepper, cut into 1" pieces

4 cups cooked brown rice

1. In a small bowl, combine the tomato paste, soy sauce, mustard, garlic, and pineapple juice. Set aside.

2. In a large skillet, heat the oil over medium-high heat. Cook the chicken, stirring constantly, for 5 minutes or until cooked through. Use a slotted spoon to transfer the chicken to a plate. Cover and keep warm.

3. Add the bell pepper to the skillet. Cook, stirring constantly, for 30 seconds. Add the chicken, pineapple chunks, and the tomato mixture. Cook, stirring, until mixture is heated through. Serve over the rice.

MAKES 4 SERVINGS

Per serving: 491 calories, 30 g protein, 74 g carbohydrates, 8 g fat, 1.5 g saturated fat, 6 g fiber, 614 mg sodium

Strawberry Cream Frostie

The riper the berries you use, the sweeter the drink. If you need a little more sweetness, add a pinch or drop of stevia. If you don't have crushed ice on hand, crush half a dozen whole cubes in the blender before you make the smoothie.

PREP TIME: 5 MINUTES ■ TOTAL TIME: 5 MINUTES

1 cup fresh or frozen strawberries

3 tablespoons half-and-half

1 tablespoon ground flaxseeds or white chia seeds

½ cup crushed ice

1. In a blender, combine the strawberries, half-and-half, and seeds. Let stand for 5 minutes.

2. Blend on the highest setting for 30 seconds.

3. Add the crushed ice. Blend on the highest setting for 1 minute.

MAKES 1 SERVING

PER SERVING: 148 calories, 4 g protein, 15 g carbohydrates, 9 g fat, 4 g saturated fat, 5 g fiber, 26 mg sodium

Roasted Edamame

Turn green soybeans into a crunchy snack.

PREP TIME: 5 MINUTES ▧ TOTAL TIME: 25 MINUTES

12 ounces thawed, shelled
  edamame
1 tablespoon fresh lime juice

2 teaspoons olive oil
1½ teaspoons smoked paprika
¼ teaspoon salt

1. Preheat the oven to 400°F.

2. In a medium bowl, combine the edamame, lime juice, oil, paprika, and salt. Spread in a single layer on a large baking sheet. Roast, stirring once, for 20 minutes, or until browned.

MAKES 4 SERVINGS (2 CUPS)

PER SERVING: 117 calories, 9 g protein, 8 g carbohydrates, 6 g fat, 0.5 saturated fat, 4 g fiber, 151 mg sodium

Paula Weiant

AGE: 50

HEIGHT: 5'7"

POUNDS LOST: 9.2—including 7.8 pounds of body fat

INCHES LOST: 13.5, including 3 inches from her waist and 3.75 inches from her hips

HEALTH UPGRADE: Her blood sugar and blood pressure fell to healthier levels; her LDL cholesterol dropped 19 points.

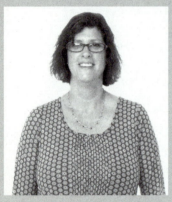

BEFORE

User-Friendly, Foolproof!

A few years ago, Paula Weiant lost 20 pounds—but then she hit a frustrating plateau. "I hung around at 150 pounds for a while," she recalls. "I wanted to lose more, but I was just stuck. I'd joined a running group and felt stronger, but I still didn't lose much weight. And since my program wasn't working, I started eating all sorts of junk food and my portions were getting bigger. If someone brought doughnuts or chocolate or cupcakes to work, I'd have some. I really needed a diet change."

It was definitely time for something new—and the 2-Day Diet was it. "I never missed the extra carbs, and I thought the amount of food you can eat is unbelievable," she says. "I love fresh salads and I'm still eating them, even though the program is over. Today, I took a salad to work with cut-up chicken, cheese, cucumbers, and an oil-and-vinegar dressing."

She and her daughter enjoyed the Taco Burgers and Tex-Mex Salad from the 5-Day Jump Start menu—and had them several times during the program. "I made the broccoli soup and the turkey panini with pesto on the weekend when there was more time to cook," she says. "On weeknights, I kept it simple and it still worked great. My daughter's still making some of the meals, like the Chocolate-Almond Smoothie, which she'll have for breakfast."

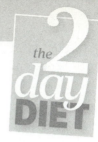

Eating well and exercising regularly soon made Paula's clothes fit loosely. But she had another goal in mind: protecting her health. "My family has a history of high blood pressure, diabetes, and heart disease," she says. "I wanted to get my numbers down and to get my total cholesterol below 200, which I accomplished on the plan. It's a personal goal of mine. And the older you get, the more you care about these things."

The 2-Day Diet's flexibility was a real plus for Paula, who fit the program into a schedule that included working two jobs (she's an administrative assistant by day, a paralegal by night) and rejoining her running group. "I made dinner when I got home from running," she says. "It was usually a variation on something in the meal plan—or just cottage cheese with fruit and nuts—but it was always satisfying." Thursdays were her "off" nights, when she enjoyed a beer and french fries with friends. "I just counted that as a day I didn't diet," she says, "and I never had a hard time getting back on track. This plan is so user-friendly that you can't mess up!"

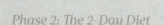

Week 2

PANTRY

- Almond extract (optional)
- Almonds, sliced natural
- Baking powder
- Baking soda
- Black pepper, ground
- Canola oil
- Cumin, ground
- Curry powder
- Honey
- Mustard, Dijon
- Mayonnaise
- Oats, quick-cooking, 1 box
- Olive oil
- Raisin bran (or other high-fiber cereal)
- Rosemary
- Sage
- Salt
- Vinegar, red wine
- Whole wheat flour

DAIRY/REFRIGERATED

- Cheese, Monterey Jack, 2 ounces
- Cheese, mozzarella, fresh, 8 ounces
- Cheese, mozzarella, part-skim, 1 pound
- Cheese, Neufchâtel, 8 ounces
- Cheese, Parmesan, grated, ½ cup
- Cheese, provolone, 2 ounces
- Cheese spread, light herbed, 4 ounces
- Cheese, Swiss, reduced-sodium, 2 ounces
- Eggs, large, 2 dozen
- Guacamole, prepared, ¼ cup
- Hummus, prepared, 10 ounces
- Milk, 1%, ½ gallon
- Shirataki noodles, 1 package (8 ounces)
- Soy milk, light, ½ gallon
- Yogurt, Greek, 2%, plain, ½ cup

MEAT, POULTRY, SEAFOOD

- Chicken breast, boneless, skinless, 5 (5 ounces each)
- Lamb shoulder or leg (or beef sirloin or tenderloin), 1 pound
- Pork tenderloin, 1 pound
- Shrimp, large, 1 pound
- Steak, sirloin, 4 (5 ounces each)
- Turkey bacon, 12 ounces
- Turkey breakfast sausage, loose, 8 ounces

FRUIT

- Apple, 1
- Banana, 1
- Blueberries, ½ pint
- Cantaloupe, 1
- Grapefruit, 1
- Lemon, 4
- Lime, 4
- Mango, 1
- Orange, 1
- Pineapple, 1
- Raspberries, ¼ cup
- Strawberries, 1 cup

VEGETABLES

- Arugula, 2 bunches
- Avocado, 1
- Basil, fresh, 1 bunch
- Broccoli, 1 bunch
- Carrots, baby, 1 bag

- Celery, 1 bunch
- Cilantro, fresh, 1 bunch
- Cucumber, 2
- Garlic, 1 head
- Green beans, 1 cup
- Lettuce, romaine hearts, 4
- Mushrooms, small, 3 containers
- Onion, red, 1
- Parsley, ¼ cup
- Red bell pepper, 2
- Salad greens, mixed, 8 cups
- Scallion, 1 bunch
- Spinach, 6 cups
- Sweet potato, 2 large
- Tomatoes, cherry, 1 pint
- Tomatoes, plum, 3
- Zucchini, 1

BREAD AND BAKED GOODS

- Bagel, whole grain, 1
- Bread, sliced, low-carb or high-fiber, 1 loaf
- Pita, whole grain, flat, 1 package

FROZEN

- Yogurt dessert, 1 container (16 ounces)

DELI

- Ham, reduced-sodium, 2 ounces

GROCERIES

- Almond meal, 1 small bag (8 ounces)
- Black beans, no-salt-added, 1 can (15–19 ounces)
- Broth, chicken or vegetable, low-fat, reduced-sodium, 3 cans (14.5 ounces each)

- Chili sauce, small bottle
- Coconut flakes, unsweetened, 1 small bag (7 ounces)
- Coconut flour, 1 small bag (16 ounces or smaller)
- Dried plums, 1 package (6 ounces)
- Mandarin oranges, 1 can (11 ounces)
- Pasta, penne, whole grain, 12 ounces
- Peanuts, unsalted, dry-roasted, ⅓ cup
- Quinoa, 1 small package (8 or 12 ounces)
- Rice, brown basmati, 1 bag (2 pounds)
- Roasted red peppers, 1 jar (16 ounces)
- Soup, lentil, reduced-sodium, 1 can (10¾ ounces)
- Soup, minestrone, reduced-sodium, 1 can (10¾ ounces)
- Sun-dried tomatoes in oil, chopped, 1 jar (8.5 ounces or smaller)
- Sunflower seeds, shelled, ¼ cup
- Tomato sauce, no-salt-added, ¼ cup
- Tomatoes, stewed, no-salt-added, 1 can (14.5 ounces)
- Tuna, 1 can (5 ounces) or pouch (2.6 ounces)
- Walnuts, chopped, 1 small bag (8 ounces)

MISCELLANEOUS

- Wooden skewers (10"), 8 (optional; only if you don't already have metal skewers)

LUNCH TAKEOUT

- 1 cup chicken rice soup
- 1 slice bread
- ½ cup three-bean salad
- 1 apple

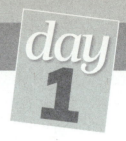

Low-Carb Day

Check what you ate or write in substitutions below.
(Asterisk indicates recipe provided later in chapter)

BREAKFAST *22 GRAMS CARBOHYDRATES*

	SUBSTITUTIONS/NOTES:
☐ Coconut-Almond Pancakes* topped with	
☐ ¼ cup 2% plain Greek yogurt mixed with stevia or Splenda, if desired	

Per serving: 488 calories, 26 g protein, 22 g carbohydrates, 36 g fat, 9 g saturated fat, 9 g fiber,
486 mg sodium

RATE YOUR HUNGER BEFORE EATING:	1 2 3 4 5 6 7 8 9 10								
RATE YOUR SATISFACTION AFTERWARD:	1 2 3 4 5 6 7 8 9 10								

LUNCH *5 GRAMS CARBOHYDRATES*

	SUBSTITUTIONS/NOTES:
☐ 2 cups mixed green salad	
☐ 4 ounces grilled chicken breast	
☐ 1 tablespoon Caesar Dressing (page 149)	
☐ 1 ounce provolone cheese	

Per serving: 398 calories, 44 g protein, 5 g carbohydrates, 22 g fat, 7 g saturated fat, 2 g fiber,
446 mg sodium

RATE YOUR HUNGER BEFORE EATING:	1 2 3 4 5 6 7 8 9 10								
RATE YOUR SATISFACTION AFTERWARD:	1 2 3 4 5 6 7 8 9 10								

DINNER *16 GRAMS CARBOHYDRATES*

SUBSTITUTIONS/NOTES:

☐ Pizza Steak,* served over
☐ ½ cup shirataki noodles
☐ 1 cup broccoli sautéed with
    1 teaspoon minced garlic in
    1 tablespoon olive oil

Per serving: 518 calories, 42 g protein, 16 g carbohydrates, 32 g fat, 8 g saturated fat, 7 g fiber,
273 mg sodium

RATE YOUR HUNGER BEFORE EATING:	1	2	3	4	5	6	7	8	9	10
RATE YOUR SATISFACTION AFTERWARD:	1	2	3	4	5	6	7	8	9	10

SNACK *7 GRAMS CARBOHYDRATES*

SUBSTITUTIONS/NOTES:

☐ 2 Deviled Eggs with Hummus*

Per serving: 242 calories, 14 g protein, 7 g carbohydrates, 18 g fat, 4 g saturated fat, 1 g fiber,
460 mg sodium

RATE YOUR HUNGER BEFORE EATING:	1	2	3	4	5	6	7	8	9	10
RATE YOUR SATISFACTION AFTERWARD:	1	2	3	4	5	6	7	8	9	10

Per day: 1,646 calories, 126 g protein, 50 g carbohydrates, 107 g fat, 29 g saturated fat, 19 g fiber,
1,665 mg sodium, 858 mg calcium, 69 IU vitamin D

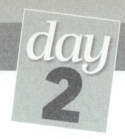
Low-Carb Day

Check what you ate or write in substitutions below.
(Asterisk indicates recipe provided later in chapter)

BREAKFAST *10 GRAMS CARBOHYDRATES*

	SUBSTITUTIONS/NOTES:
☐ 2 eggs, any style	
☐ 2 slices turkey bacon	
☐ ½ grapefruit	

Per serving: 387 calories, 18 g protein, 10 g carbohydrates, 30 g fat, 10 g saturated fat, 1 g fiber, 672 mg sodium

RATE YOUR HUNGER BEFORE EATING:	1 2 3 4 5 6 7 8 9 10
RATE YOUR SATISFACTION AFTERWARD:	1 2 3 4 5 6 7 8 9 10

LUNCH *14 GRAMS CARBOHYDRATES*

	SUBSTITUTIONS/NOTES:
☐ Roast Beef and Guacamole in Lettuce Boats*	
☐ 1 ounce Monterey Jack cheese	

Per serving: 667 calories, 62 g protein, 14 g carbohydrates, 40 g fat, 19 g saturated fat, 3 g fiber, 834 mg sodium

RATE YOUR HUNGER BEFORE EATING:	1 2 3 4 5 6 7 8 9 10
RATE YOUR SATISFACTION AFTERWARD:	1 2 3 4 5 6 7 8 9 10

DINNER *16 GRAMS CARBOHYDRATES*

☐ 2 cups mixed green salad with

☐ 1 tablespoon Caesar Dressing (page 149)

☐ Chicken Breasts Stuffed with Spinach and Sun-Dried Tomatoes*

☐ 1 cup zucchini, sautéed in

☐ 2 teaspoons olive oil

☐ ½ cup shirataki noodles with

☐ 2 teaspoons olive oil and

☐ 1 tablespoon Parmesan cheese

Per serving: 664 calories, 45 g protein, 16 g carbohydrates, 49 g fat, 11 g saturated fat, 7 g fiber, 637 mg sodium

SUBSTITUTIONS/NOTES:

RATE YOUR HUNGER BEFORE EATING:	1	2	3	4	5	6	7	8	9	10
RATE YOUR SATISFACTION AFTERWARD:	1	2	3	4	5	6	7	8	9	10

SNACK *10 GRAMS CARBOHYDRATES*

☐ 1 cup cucumber slices spread with

☐ 2 tablespoons hummus mixed with

☐ 1 tablespoon marinated chopped sun-dried tomatoes

Per serving: 82 calories, 3 g protein, 10 g carbohydrates, 4 g fat, 1 g saturated fat, 3 g fiber, 139 mg sodium

SUBSTITUTIONS/NOTES:

RATE YOUR HUNGER BEFORE EATING:	1	2	3	4	5	6	7	8	9	10
RATE YOUR SATISFACTION AFTERWARD:	1	2	3	4	5	6	7	8	9	10

Per day: 1,800 calories, 128 g protein, 50 g carbohydrates, 124 g fat, 40 g saturated fat, 14 g fiber, 2,282 mg sodium, 716 mg calcium, 110 IU vitamin D

Regular-Carb Day

day
3

Check what you ate or write in substitutions below.
(Asterisk indicates recipe provided later in chapter)

BREAKFAST

SUBSTITUTIONS/NOTES:

☐ ¾ cup high-fiber cereal

☐ 1 cup 1% milk

☐ 1 orange

Per serving: 254 calories, 12 g protein, 65 g carbohydrates, 4 g fat, 2 g saturated fat, 24 g fiber,
265 mg sodium

RATE YOUR HUNGER BEFORE EATING: 1 2 3 4 5 6 7 8 9 10
RATE YOUR SATISFACTION AFTERWARD: 1 2 3 4 5 6 7 8 9 10

LUNCH

SUBSTITUTIONS/NOTES:

☐ 2 cups spinach and

☐ ½ cup mushrooms with

☐ 1 serving Rosemary Balsamic
  Vinaigrette (page 107)

☐ Lemon-Quinoa Salad with Sunflower
  Seeds*

Per serving: 569 calories, 11 g protein, 43 g carbohydrates, 41 g fat, 5 g saturated fat, 7 g fiber,
352 mg sodium

RATE YOUR HUNGER BEFORE EATING: 1 2 3 4 5 6 7 8 9 10
RATE YOUR SATISFACTION AFTERWARD: 1 2 3 4 5 6 7 8 9 10

DINNER

☐ Pork Medallions in Sage Broth*

☐ 1 medium sweet potato, baked

☐ 2 cups arugula or spinach sautéed with

☐ 1 teaspoon minced garlic in

☐ 1 tablespoon olive oil

☐ 1 cup pineapple cubes

Per serving: 497 calories, 28 g protein, 50 g carbohydrates, 22 g fat, 4 g saturated fat, 7 g fiber, 255 mg sodium

SUBSTITUTIONS/NOTES:

RATE YOUR HUNGER BEFORE EATING:	1	2	3	4	5	6	7	8	9	10
RATE YOUR SATISFACTION AFTERWARD:	1	2	3	4	5	6	7	8	9	10

SNACK

☐ ½ cup frozen yogurt with

☐ 2 tablespoons chopped dried plums and

☐ 2 tablespoons sliced natural almonds

Per serving: 211 calories, 5 g protein, 30 g carbohydrates, 9 g fat, 2 g saturated fat, 3 g fiber, 57 mg sodium

SUBSTITUTIONS/NOTES:

RATE YOUR HUNGER BEFORE EATING:	1	2	3	4	5	6	7	8	9	10
RATE YOUR SATISFACTION AFTERWARD:	1	2	3	4	5	6	7	8	9	10

Per day: 1,531 calories, 56 g protein, 189 g carbohydrates, 76 g fat, 14 g saturated fat, 41 g fiber, 928 mg sodium, 873 mg calcium, 17 IU vitamin D

Regular-Carb Day

Check what you ate or write in substitutions below.
(Asterisk indicates recipe provided later in chapter)

BREAKFAST

☐ ½ whole wheat bagel spread with

☐ 2 tablespoons Neufchâtel cream cheese

☐ ¼ cantaloupe

Per serving: 257 calories, 9 g protein, 38 g carbohydrates, 7 g fat, 4 g saturated fat, 6 g fiber, 362 mg sodium

SUBSTITUTIONS/NOTES:

RATE YOUR HUNGER BEFORE EATING:	1	2	3	4	5	6	7	8	9	10
RATE YOUR SATISFACTION AFTERWARD:	1	2	3	4	5	6	7	8	9	10

LUNCH

☐ 2 cups mixed green salad with

☐ 1 serving Lime Vinaigrette (page 111)

☐ Sweet Potato Soup with Tomato and Lime*

☐ 1 slice low-carb or high-fiber bread topped with

☐ 1 ounce Cheddar cheese, melted

Per serving: 648 calories, 21 g protein, 48 g carbohydrates, 44 g fat, 11 g saturated fat, 11 g fiber, 664 mg sodium

SUBSTITUTIONS/NOTES:

RATE YOUR HUNGER BEFORE EATING:	1	2	3	4	5	6	7	8	9	10
RATE YOUR SATISFACTION AFTERWARD:	1	2	3	4	5	6	7	8	9	10

DINNER

	SUBSTITUTIONS/NOTES:
☐ 1 cucumber and ½ red onion, sliced, with	
☐ 1 tablespoon ranch dressing	
☐ Meat and Veggie Kebabs*	
☐ 1 cup cooked brown basmati rice	

Per serving: 541 calories, 31 g protein, 56 g carbohydrates, 23 g fat, 4.5 g saturated fat, 7 g fiber,
649 mg sodium

RATE YOUR HUNGER BEFORE EATING: 1   2   3   4   5   6   7   8   9   10
RATE YOUR SATISFACTION AFTERWARD: 1   2   3   4   5   6   7   8   9   10

SNACK

	SUBSTITUTIONS/NOTES:
☐ 1 cup baby carrots and	
☐ 2 celery sticks with	
☐ ⅓ cup hummus mixed with	
☐ 2 tablespoons sun-dried tomatoes	

Per serving: 183 calories, 8 g protein, 20 g carbohydrates, 9 g fat, 1 g saturated fat, 8 g fiber,
439 mg sodium

RATE YOUR HUNGER BEFORE EATING: 1   2   3   4   5   6   7   8   9   10
RATE YOUR SATISFACTION AFTERWARD: 1   2   3   4   5   6   7   8   9   10

Per day: 1,629 calories, 68 g protein, 163 g carbohydrates, 83 g fat, 21 g saturated fat, 32 g fiber,
2,115 mg sodium, 681 mg calcium, 12 IU vitamin D

Regular-Carb Day

Check what you ate or write in substitutions below.
(Asterisk indicates recipe provided later in chapter)

BREAKFAST

SUBSTITUTIONS/NOTES:

☐ Sausage Strata*

☐ 1 cup strawberries, sliced

☐ 1 cup 1% low-fat milk

Per serving: 491 calories, 37 g protein, 40 g carbohydrates, 21 g fat, 8 g saturated fat, 7 g fiber, 649 mg sodium

RATE YOUR HUNGER BEFORE EATING:	1	2	3	4	5	6	7	8	9	10
RATE YOUR SATISFACTION AFTERWARD:	1	2	3	4	5	6	7	8	9	10

LUNCH

SUBSTITUTIONS/NOTES:

☐ Tuna salad or chicken salad sandwich

☐ ½ cup baby carrots

☐ 1 apple

Per serving: 376 calories, 25 g protein, 53 g carbohydrates, 10 g fat, 2 g saturated fat, 12 g fiber, 701 mg sodium

RATE YOUR HUNGER BEFORE EATING:	1	2	3	4	5	6	7	8	9	10
RATE YOUR SATISFACTION AFTERWARD:	1	2	3	4	5	6	7	8	9	10

DINNER

	SUBSTITUTIONS/NOTES:

☐ Black Bean Pita Pizza*

☐ ½ cup fresh or drained, canned
  pineapple chunks

Per serving: 542 calories, 20 g protein, 70 g carbohydrates, 21 g fat, 7 g saturated fat, 11 g fiber,
768 mg sodium

RATE YOUR HUNGER BEFORE EATING:	1 2 3 4 5 6 7 8 9 10
RATE YOUR SATISFACTION AFTERWARD:	1 2 3 4 5 6 7 8 9 10

SNACK

	SUBSTITUTIONS/NOTES:

☐ 2 ounces Swiss cheese

☐ 2 tablespoons nuts

Per serving: 318 calories, 19 g protein, 6 g carbohydrates, 25 g fat, 11 g saturated fat, 2 g fiber,
109 mg sodium

RATE YOUR HUNGER BEFORE EATING:	1 2 3 4 5 6 7 8 9 10
RATE YOUR SATISFACTION AFTERWARD:	1 2 3 4 5 6 7 8 9 10

Per day: 1,728 calories, 101 g protein, 169 g carbohydrates, 76 g fat, 27 g saturated fat, 31 g fiber,
2,227 mg sodium, 1,615 mg calcium, 118 IU vitamin D

Regular-Carb Day

Check what you ate or write in substitutions below.
(Asterisk indicates recipe provided later in chapter)

BREAKFAST

□ 1 cup cooked oatmeal

□ 1 banana

□ 2 tablespoons chopped nuts

□ 1 cup 1% milk

Per serving: 451 calories, 18 g protein, 70 g carbohydrates, 13 g fat, 3 g saturated fat, 9 g fiber,
118 mg sodium

SUBSTITUTIONS/NOTES:

RATE YOUR HUNGER BEFORE EATING: 1   2   3   4   5   6   7   8   9   10
RATE YOUR SATISFACTION AFTERWARD: 1   2   3   4   5   6   7   8   9   10

LUNCH

□ 1 cup chicken and wild rice soup

□ 1 slice low-carb bread

□ ½ cup three-bean salad

□ 1 apple

Per serving: 325 calories, 12 g protein, 64 g carbohydrates, 4 g fat, 0.5 g saturated fat, 11 g fiber,
1,332 mg sodium

SUBSTITUTIONS/NOTES:

RATE YOUR HUNGER BEFORE EATING: 1   2   3   4   5   6   7   8   9   10
RATE YOUR SATISFACTION AFTERWARD: 1   2   3   4   5   6   7   8   9   10

DINNER

	SUBSTITUTIONS/NOTES:
☐ Caribbean Chili-Lime Shrimp with Peanuts*	
☐ 1 cup brown basmati rice	
☐ 1 cup steamed green beans	
☐ ½ cup mango cubes	

Per serving: 508 calories, 30 g protein, 71 g carbohydrates, 14 g fat, 2 g saturated fat, 9 g fiber, 226 mg sodium

RATE YOUR HUNGER BEFORE EATING:	1 2 3 4 5 6 7 8 9 10
RATE YOUR SATISFACTION AFTERWARD:	1 2 3 4 5 6 7 8 9 10

SNACK

	SUBSTITUTIONS/NOTES:
☐ 1 ounce chocolate with	
☐ 12 almonds, pecans, or walnuts	

Per serving: 244 calories, 5 g protein, 18 g carbohydrates, 19 g fat, 7 g saturated fat, 4 g fiber, 0 mg sodium

RATE YOUR HUNGER BEFORE EATING:	1 2 3 4 5 6 7 8 9 10
RATE YOUR SATISFACTION AFTERWARD:	1 2 3 4 5 6 7 8 9 10

Per day: 1,528 calories, 66 g protein, 224 g carbohydrates, 50 g fat, 12 g saturated fat, 33 g fiber, 1,676 mg sodium, 663 mg calcium, 2 IU vitamin D

Regular-Carb Day

Check what you ate or write in substitutions below.
(Asterisk indicates recipe provided later in chapter)

BREAKFAST

☐ Oatmeal Breakfast Bread*

☐ 2 tablespoons almond or peanut butter

☐ ½ cup blueberries

Per serving: 472 calories, 12 g protein, 49 g carbohydrates, 28 g fat, 4 g saturated fat, 7 g fiber, 508 mg sodium

SUBSTITUTIONS/NOTES:

RATE YOUR HUNGER BEFORE EATING:	1	2	3	4	5	6	7	8	9	10
RATE YOUR SATISFACTION AFTERWARD:	1	2	3	4	5	6	7	8	9	10

LUNCH

☐ 1 cup lentil soup

☐ 2 cups spinach leaves tossed with

☐ 1 tablespoon olive oil,

☐ ½ cup mandarin orange sections,

☐ 2 tablespoons chopped almonds, and

☐ 2 tablespoons finely chopped cilantro or parsley (if desired)

☐ 2 ounces thinly sliced reduced-sodium ham

Per serving: 434 calories, 23 g protein, 34 g carbohydrates, 26 g fat, 3 g saturated fat, 13 g fiber, 1,071 mg sodium

SUBSTITUTIONS/NOTES:

RATE YOUR HUNGER BEFORE EATING:	1	2	3	4	5	6	7	8	9	10
RATE YOUR SATISFACTION AFTERWARD:	1	2	3	4	5	6	7	8	9	10

DINNER

	SUBSTITUTIONS/NOTES:
☐ 2 cups mixed green salad with	
☐ 1 recipe Rosemary Balsamic Vinaigrette (page 107)	
☐ Penne Pasta with Roast Peppers and Mozzarella*	

Per serving: 703 calories, 21 g protein, 44 g carbohydrates, 50 g fat, 14 g saturated fat, 9 g fiber, 485 mg sodium

RATE YOUR HUNGER BEFORE EATING:	1	2	3	4	5	6	7	8	9	10
RATE YOUR SATISFACTION AFTERWARD:	1	2	3	4	5	6	7	8	9	10

SNACK

	SUBSTITUTIONS/NOTES:
☐ 1 cup 2% plain Greek yogurt blended with	
☐ ½ tablespoon cocoa powder and	
☐ 1 packet stevia or Splenda	

Per serving: 140 calories, 18 g protein, 11 g carbohydrates, 4 g fat, 3 g saturated fat, 1 g fiber, 66 mg sodium

RATE YOUR HUNGER BEFORE EATING:	1	2	3	4	5	6	7	8	9	10
RATE YOUR SATISFACTION AFTERWARD:	1	2	3	4	5	6	7	8	9	10

Per day: 1, 749 calories, 73 g protein, 138 g carbohydrates, 109 g fat, 24 g saturated fat, 29 g fiber, 2,129 mg sodium, 909 mg calcium, 6 IU vitamin D

Coconut-Almond Pancakes

Yes, you can have pancakes on a low-carb day!

PREP TIME: 10 MINUTES ■ TOTAL TIME: 20 MINUTES

½ cup almond meal

¼ cup coconut flour

¼ cup unsweetened shredded coconut

¼ teaspoon salt

4 egg whites

1 cup 1% milk

¼ teaspoon almond extract

Canola oil

1. In a large bowl, combine the almond meal, coconut flour, shredded coconut, and salt.

2. In a small, clean glass bowl, beat the egg whites with a hand mixer until stiff peaks form.

3. Stir the milk, almond extract, and beaten egg whites gently into the flour mixture.

4. Heat the oil in a griddle or skillet over medium heat. Pour the batter onto the cooking surface, using ½ cup per pancake. Cook 3 to 4 minutes, carefully turning once, or until lightly browned on both sides.

MAKES 2 SERVINGS (2 PANCAKES PER SERVING)

PER SERVING: 451 calories, 21 g protein, 20 g carbohydrates, 34 g fat, 9 g saturated fat, 9 g fiber, 467 mg sodium

Sausage Strata

A strata is a casserole that is assembled the night before, so all you have to do is pop it in the oven the next morning. This recipe calls for loose sausage, but if you can only find links, simply remove the casings. Take the strata out of the refrigerator 30 minutes before baking.

PREP TIME: 20 MINUTES PLUS CHILLING TIME
TOTAL TIME: 1 HOUR 5 MINUTES PLUS CHILLING AND STANDING TIME

6 slices low-carb bread

1 tablespoon olive oil

8 ounces loose turkey or pork breakfast sausage

1½ cups shredded part-skim mozzarella cheese

2 plum tomatoes, finely chopped

6 eggs

2 cups 1% milk

1 tablespoon Dijon mustard

1. Coat an 11" × 7" baking pan with cooking spray. Line with overlapping slices of bread.

2. Heat the oil in a large skillet over medium heat. Add the sausage and cook, stirring often, for 5 minutes, or until no longer pink. Spoon the sausage over the bread. Sprinkle with the cheese and tomatoes.

3. In a medium bowl, combine the eggs, milk, and mustard. Pour evenly over the bread. Cover and refrigerate overnight.

4. Preheat the oven to 350°F. Bake for 45 minutes, or until a wooden pick inserted in the center comes out clean. Let stand for 15 minutes before slicing and serving.

MAKES 6 SERVINGS

PER SERVING: 337 calories, 28 g protein, 15 g carbohydrates, 18 g fat, 6 g saturated fat, 3 g fiber, 540 mg sodium

Oatmeal Breakfast Bread

For a lighter loaf, substitute 1 cup of whole grain pastry flour for 1 cup of the whole wheat flour.

PREP TIME: 15 MINUTES ■ TOTAL TIME: 55 MINUTES PLUS STANDING TIME

1¼ cups low-fat plain yogurt
1 cup quick oats
2 eggs
¼ cup honey
⅓ cup olive oil

2 cups whole wheat flour
2 teaspoons baking powder
½ teaspoon baking soda
¾ teaspoon salt
½ cup diced dried plums (prunes), optional

1. Preheat the oven to 350°F. Coat a 9" × 5" loaf pan with cooking spray.

2. In a large bowl, combine the yogurt and oats. Let stand for 10 minutes.

3. Stir in the eggs, honey, and oil.

4. In a medium bowl, combine the flour, baking powder, baking soda, and salt. Stir into the oat mixture. Stir in the plums (if using).

5. Bake for 35 to 40 minutes, or until a toothpick inserted in the center comes out clean. Let cool for 30 minutes before slicing and serving.

MAKES 10 SERVINGS

PER SERVING: 231 calories, 7 g protein, 32 g carbohydrates, 10 g fat, 2 g saturated fat, 4 g fiber, 366 mg sodium

Baked Egg and Ham Cup

A tasty low-carb breakfast for a busy weekday morning. Pop it in the oven while you finish getting ready for work!

PREP TIME: 5 MINUTES ■ TOTAL TIME: 20 MINUTES

1 thin slice reduced-sodium ham (about ½ ounce)

2 eggs

2 tablespoons grated Parmesan cheese

1. Preheat the oven to 375°F. Coat an 8-ounce custard cup with cooking spray.

2. Line the cup with the ham slice.

3. Break the eggs and pour them into the ham and sprinkle with the cheese.

4. Bake for 15 minutes or until the white is set.

MAKES 1 SERVING

PER SERVING: 180 calories, 17 g protein, 1 g carbohydrates, 12 g fat, 4 g saturated fat, 0 g fiber, 333 mg sodium

Roast Beef and Guacamole in Lettuce Boats

Use leftover beef from the Beef and Vegetable Roast dinner (page 155).

PREP TIME: 10 MINUTES ■ TOTAL TIME: 10 MINUTES

4 large leaves romaine lettuce

1 cup diced cooked roast beef

¼ cup guacamole

¼ cup salsa

1 scallion, thinly sliced

Top each lettuce leaf with ¼ cup roast beef and one-fourth of the guacamole, salsa, and scallion slices. Roll and enjoy!

MAKES 1 SERVING

PER SERVING: 561 calories, 55 g protein, 14 g carbohydrates, 31 g fat, 13 g saturated fat, 3 g fiber, 683 mg sodium

Lemon-Quinoa Salad with Sunflower Seeds

Quinoa is a quick-cooking grain rich in fiber and protein.

PREP TIME: 10 MINUTES ■ TOTAL TIME: 10 MINUTES

2 cups cherry tomatoes, sliced in half

1 small cucumber sliced lengthwise, seeds removed, and sliced thinly

2 scallions, sliced

¼ cup fresh lemon juice

2 tablespoons olive oil

½ teaspoon salt

3 cups cooked quinoa

¼ cup sunflower seeds

1. Place the tomatoes, cucumber, and scallions in a large bowl.

2. In a small bowl, combine the lemon juice, oil, and salt.

3. Add the quinoa and sunflower seeds to the large bowl. Drizzle with the dressing and toss to combine.

MAKES 4 SERVINGS

PER SERVING: 290 calories, 9 g protein, 37 g carbohydrates, 13 g fat, 1.5 g saturated fat, 6 g fiber, 306 mg sodium

Sweet Potato Soup
with Tomato and Lime

If you don't have leftover sweet potato on hand, finely chop a fresh one and simmer it with the broth for an extra minute or two until very tender, then mash it right in the pot with a potato masher or fork.

PREP TIME: 15 MINUTES ■ TOTAL TIME: 35 MINUTES

1 tablespoon olive oil

1 onion, finely chopped

2 cloves garlic, finely chopped

1 teaspoon curry powder or cumin

2 cups mashed sweet potato
(1 large)

2 cans (14.5 ounces each) low-fat, reduced-sodium chicken or vegetable broth

1 large tomato, finely chopped

2 tablespoons fresh lime juice

½ cup finely chopped cilantro

1. Heat the oil in a large saucepan over medium heat. Add the onion and cook for 4 minutes. Add the garlic and curry powder or cumin. Cook for 1 minute.

2. Add the sweet potato and broth. Heat to a boil. Reduce the heat to medium-low and simmer for 10 minutes, or until heated through.

3. Stir in the tomato and lime juice. Simmer for 1 minute. Sprinkle with the cilantro and serve.

MAKES 4 SERVINGS (6 CUPS)

PER SERVING: 213 calories, 8 g protein, 35 g carbohydrates, 5 g fat, 1 g saturated fat, 6 g fiber, 501 mg sodium

Chicken Noodle Soup with Spinach and Basil

A new twist on a classic lunchtime favorite. To shred the basil and spinach leaves, stack a few leaves on top of each other and roll up tightly from a long side. Thinly slice crosswise into shreds.

PREP TIME: 15 MINUTES ■ TOTAL TIME: 25 MINUTES

1 package (8 ounces) shirataki spaghetti noodles (4 ounces after draining and rinsing)

2 tablespoons olive oil

1½ pounds boneless, skinless chicken breast, cut into bite-size pieces

2 scallions, thinly sliced

2 cans (14.5 ounces each) low-fat, reduced-sodium chicken broth

4 cups spinach leaves, shredded

1 cup basil leaves, shredded

1 tablespoon fresh lemon juice

1. Cook the shirataki noodles according to the package directions. Drain and set aside.

2. Meanwhile, in a large saucepan, heat the oil. Cook the chicken and scallion for 5 minutes, or until lightly browned. Add the broth and bring to a simmer over medium heat. Add the spinach, basil, and lemon juice. Simmer 4 minutes, or until the spinach is wilted and the chicken is cooked through.

3. Add the noodles to the soup

MAKES 4 SERVINGS

PER SERVING: 278 calories, 38 g protein, 5 g carbohydrates, 11 g fat, 2 g saturated fat, 2 g fiber, 688 mg sodium

Pizza Steak

Now you can enjoy the flavor of pizza, even on low-carb days!

PREP TIME: 10 MINUTES ▨ TOTAL TIME: 20 MINUTES

1 tablespoon olive oil

4 boneless strip steaks (5 ounces each)

1 can (14.5 ounces) no-salt-added stewed tomatoes

½ cup shredded part-skim mozzarella cheese

¼ cup grated Parmesan cheese

1. Heat the oil in a large skillet over medium heat. Add the steaks and brown for 1 to 2 minutes on each side.

2. Add the tomatoes and simmer for 5 minutes.

3. Top with the cheeses and cook until melted.

MAKES 4 SERVINGS

PER SERVING: 348 calories, 38 g protein, 8 g carbohydrates, 17 g fat, 6 g saturated fat, 2 g fiber, 233 mg sodium

Chicken Breasts Stuffed with Spinach and Sun-Dried Tomatoes

You can substitute feta or Swiss cheese for the mozzarella and use half of a 10-ounce package of frozen and thawed chopped spinach instead of fresh.

PREP TIME: 15 MINUTES ■ TOTAL TIME: 30 MINUTES

2 cups spinach leaves, coarsely chopped

4 cups boiling water

4 boneless, skinless chicken breasts (about 1¼ pounds total)

¼ cup chopped sun-dried tomatoes, packed in oil

4 ounces part-skim mozzarella cheese, shredded

2 tablespoons olive oil

1 tablespoon red wine vinegar

1. Place the spinach in a colander in the sink. Pour the boiling water over the spinach to wilt. Drain well.

2. Place the chicken breasts between 2 sheets of waxed paper and use the bottom of a heavy skillet or saucepan to pound to ¼" thickness.

3. Divide the spinach, tomatoes, and cheese evenly over the breasts to within ½" of the edges. Roll up each breast from one short end. Fasten with a wooden pick.

4. Heat the oil in a large skillet over medium heat. Add the chicken breasts and cook, turning occasionally, for 6 minutes, or until browned on all sides. Cover and cook for 6 to 8 minutes, or until a thermometer inserted into the center of a breast registers 165°F and the juices run clear.

5. Transfer the chicken breasts to a platter and cover to keep warm. Add the vinegar to the skillet and cook for 10 seconds, scraping up any brown bits from the bottom of the pan. Drizzle over the chicken and serve.

MAKES 4 SERVINGS

PER SERVING: 323 calories, 38 g protein, 3 g carbohydrates, 18 g fat, 6 g saturated fat, 0 g fiber, 417 mg sodium

Pork Medallions in Sage Broth

Sage and pork, the perfect marriage of flavors!

PREP TIME: 5 MINUTES ■ TOTAL TIME: 10 MINUTES

1 pound pork tenderloin

1 tablespoon olive oil

1 cup fat-free chicken broth

½ teaspoon dried sage, crumbled

1. Cut the pork tenderloin into ¾"-thick slices.

2. Heat the oil in a large skillet over medium-high heat. Add the pork and cook until browned on both sides.

3. Add the broth and sage. Lower the heat and simmer for 1 to 2 minutes, or until a thermometer inserted in the center of a medallion registers 160°F and the juices run clear.

MAKES 4 SERVINGS

PER SERVING: 170 calories, 24 g protein, 0 g carbohydrates, 8 g fat, 2 g saturated fat, 0 g fiber, 172 mg sodium

Meat and Veggie Kebabs

If you use disposable wooden skewers for your kebabs, soak them in water for 30 minutes before cooking to prevent burning. If you're a garlic lover, add 3 or 4 chopped cloves to the marinade.

PREP TIME: 20 MINUTES PLUS MARINATING ▪ TOTAL TIME: 35 MINUTES PLUS MARINATING

2 tablespoons olive oil

2 tablespoons red wine vinegar

1 tablespoon dried rosemary, crushed

¾ teaspoon salt

1 pound lean lamb shoulder or leg, or beef sirloin or tenderloin, cut into 1" cubes (32 cubes)

1 red onion, halved, each half cut into 12 pieces

24 small mushrooms, stemmed, or 12 large mushrooms, stemmed and halved

1 red bell pepper, halved, each half cut into 12 pieces

1. In a large bowl, combine the oil, vinegar, rosemary, and salt. Add the lamb or beef, onion, mushrooms, and pepper and toss to coat. Marinate at room temperature for 30 minutes or in the refrigerator for at least 1 hour.

2. Preheat the broiler. Line a broiler pan with aluminum foil.

3. On 8 skewers, thread alternate pieces of lamb or beef, onion, mushroom, and pepper until the skewers are filled, starting and ending with cubes of meat. Place the skewers on the lined broiler pan.

4. Broil 4" from the heat source for 5 minutes, turning once, for medium-rare, or until desired doneness.

MAKES 4 SERVINGS (2 SKEWERS EACH)

PER SERVING: 248 calories, 25 g protein, 7 g carbohydrates, 13 g fat, 3 g saturated fat, 2 g fiber, 521 mg sodium

Black Bean Pita Pizza

Beans give this pizza a flavorful and filling boost of fiber.

PREP TIME: 5 MINUTES ■ TOTAL TIME: 10 MINUTES

1 whole grain pita

2 teaspoons olive oil

¼ cup no-salt-added tomato sauce

⅓ cup no-salt-added black beans

¼ cup shredded Monterey Jack cheese

1 tablespoon finely chopped cilantro (optional)

1. On a small baking sheet, position the pita and brush with the oil.

2. Top with the tomato sauce, beans, and cheese.

3. Heat under the broiler or in a toaster oven until heated through and the cheese melts. Top with the cilantro (if using).

MAKES 1 SERVING

PER SERVING: 502 calories 19 g protein, 60 g carbohydrates, 20 g fat, 7 g saturated fat, 10 g fiber, 766 mg sodium

Penne Pasta with Roasted Peppers and Mozzarella

Dig into an Italian-inspired comfort food bursting with the sunny flavors of basil and sun-dried tomato.

PREP TIME: 10 MINUTES ■ TOTAL TIME: 15 MINUTES

12 ounces whole grain penne pasta

½ cup chopped roasted red peppers

8 ounces fresh mozzarella, finely chopped

½ cup finely chopped fresh basil

¼ cup finely chopped sun-dried tomatoes

¼ cup grated Parmesan cheese

2 tablespoons olive oil

1. Cook the penne according to package directions.

2. In a large bowl, add the pasta and toss with the peppers, mozzarella, basil, tomatoes, Parmesan, and oil.

MAKES 4 SERVINGS

PER SERVING: 422 calories, 19 g protein, 37 g carbohydrates, 22 g fat, 10 g saturated fat, 6 g fiber, 442 mg sodium

Caribbean Chili-Lime Shrimp with Peanuts

The secret ingredient in a recipe full of surprise flavors? Sweet honey.

PREP TIME: 5 MINUTES ▪ TOTAL TIME: 10 MINUTES

1 pound large shrimp, shelled and deveined

1 tablespoon olive oil

2 tablespoons fresh lime juice

1 tablespoon chili sauce

1 tablespoon honey

⅓ cup unsalted dry-roasted peanuts

1. In a large skillet over medium heat, cook the shrimp in the oil, stirring, for 3 minutes.

2. Add the lime juice, chili sauce, honey, and peanuts. Cook for 1 minute, then serve.

MAKES 4 SERVINGS

PER SERVING: 228 calories, 23 g protein, 9 g carbohydrates, 11 g fat, 2 g saturated fat, 1 g fiber, 223 mg sodium

Deviled Eggs with Hummus

Take these to the next picnic or savor as a snack at home.

PREP TIME: 10 MINUTES ▪ TOTAL TIME: 10 MINUTES

6 hard-cooked eggs, halved lengthwise

⅓ cup garlic-flavored hummus

2 tablespoons fresh lemon juice

1 tablespoon olive oil

¼ teaspoon salt

1. Remove the yolks from the eggs and mash with the hummus, lemon juice, oil, and salt.

2. Spoon the mixture back into the eggs. Refrigerate until ready to eat.

MAKES 6 SERVINGS (12 HALVES)

PER SERVING: 121 calories, 7 g protein, 4 g carbohydrates, 9 g fat, 2 g saturated fat, 0 g fiber, 230 mg sodium

Sara Phillips

AGE: 64

HEIGHT: 5'7"

POUNDS LOST: 16.6

INCHES LOST: 15, including 5 inches from her waist and 3.5 inches from her hips

HEALTH UPGRADE: Lower blood sugar and blood pressure; healthier triglycerides.

"I Lost More Than 16 Pounds!"

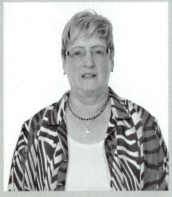

BEFORE

Sara Phillips bought new summer clothes just before starting the 2-Day Diet. "Now I have a problem," she says with a laugh. "I have to take them to the tailor and have them altered. I'm down at least one size!"

An executive administrative assistant at a nature conservancy, Sara gets to work early, so she never has much time to cook in the morning. But on the 2-Day Diet, that was no problem. "I'd make hard-cooked eggs in advance, peel them, then eat them on the way to work," she says. "On regular-carb days, I had a banana with peanut butter. I found meals and food that fit my schedule."

Making choices at the supermarket, she says, is a more enlightened experience now. "This plan changed my life when it comes to food shopping," she says. "The first thing I do now is look to see how many carbs a food has before I buy it. Even some healthy-looking cereals have a lot of carbs thanks to added sugars—so I've switched to types that are less sweetened and have fewer carbs in a serving. I compare carbs all the time now."

Sara got her exercise walking her three dogs—a standard poodle, a miniature poodle, and a miniature schnauzer. "I walk my big dog, then the two little ones," she says. "They keep me active." She's proof that the program works even if you can't follow the whole 2-Day Diet Workout. "With two torn rotator cuffs in my shoulders, a torn meniscus in my knee, a bone spur, and a heel injury, I can't do a lot

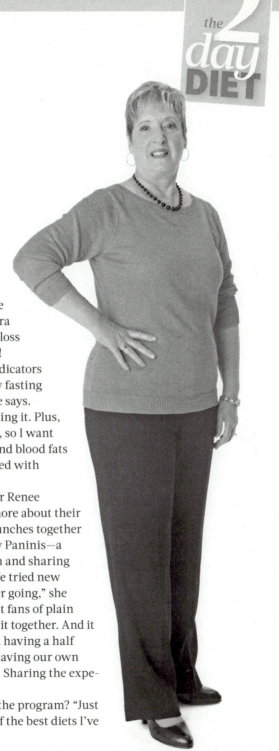

of heavy-duty exercise—but I can put on my knee brace and take a walk or ride my exercise bike," she says. Despite these limitations, Sara was happy when her final weight loss tallied up to more than 16 pounds!

Improvements in key health indicators made her happy, too. "I'm glad my fasting blood sugar level came down," she says. "My doctor and I have been watching it. Plus, there's heart disease in my family, so I want to make sure my blood pressure and blood fats are also good. The diet really helped with those."

Sara teamed up with co-worker Renee Guzenski for the program (read more about their story on page 11). The duo made lunches together in the office, cooking their Turkey Paninis—a favorite—in the office toaster oven and sharing snacks like cheese and apples. "We tried new foods together and kept each other going," she says. "Honestly, at first we weren't fans of plain yogurt, but we could laugh about it together. And it was a big day when we went from having a half apple each for our snack to each having our own apple once we'd lost some weight. Sharing the experience made it really fun."

Her advice to readers starting the program? "Just try it," she says. "I think it's one of the best diets I've ever been on."

fast and easy meals—
At Home and Away

The 2-Day Diet is all about flexibility—not just when it comes to choosing which days to go low-carb or when to exercise. This plan's versatility also means that if you don't want to cook, don't like following recipes, want to eat out, or need to grab a quick bite on the road, you can, without falling off the plan.

Our test panelists loved this feature—and said that the ability to work the plan into almost any eating situation was another key to their dramatic pounds-off and inches-off success. In this chapter, you'll discover the easiest ways to eat on the plan, with options including mix-and-match meal charts for low-carb and regular-carb days, lists of easy-to-throw-together meals and snacks, and a guide to great meal choices at leading fast-food and casual-dining chains.

The good news: Whether you're looking for a meal in minutes or want to branch out and cook with new ingredients, whether you're off for a festive night out or need to find lunch at the next fast-food drive-thru, you can do it deliciously the 2-Day Diet way. You can even fit in favorites like a hamburger and fries, the occasional ice-cream cone, shrimp scampi, wrap sandwiches, steak, fancy salads, Mexican dishes, and Asian-inspired stir-fries.

FAST AND EASY LOW-CARB MEALS AT HOME

No time to follow a recipe? Looking for 1-serving meals? No problem. We've got you covered, with five options each for breakfast, lunch, and dinner—all clocking in at about 15 grams of net carbs.

Breakfast

1. Hearty eggs and toast: Cook $1/2$ cup cooked spinach and 1 cup sliced raw mushrooms in 2 teaspoons olive oil, then add 3 beaten eggs and scramble. Top with 2 tablespoons shredded part-skim mozzarella cheese. Enjoy with 1 slice toast—choose a reduced-carb bread such as Pepperidge Farm Carb Style, or have half of a Thomas' 100% Whole Wheat Breakfast Thins Round or other bread with 11 or fewer grams of carbs per slice.

2. Yogurt delight: Top 1 cup 0% plain Greek yogurt with 1 tablespoon sliced almonds. Pair with $1/8$ of a small cantaloupe. If you prefer sweeter yogurt, first mix in a little stevia.

3. Huevos rancheros: Scramble 2 eggs, top with 2 tablespoons shredded low-fat cheese and 1 to 2 tablespoons salsa. Serve on a warm low-carb tortilla (look for one with 10 or fewer grams of carbs).

4. Scrambled or fried eggs with "hash browns": Enjoy 2 eggs cooked any style. Create low-carb "hash browns" by grating $1/2$ cup jicama (a vegetable available in the supermarket produce section), then cooking it with chopped onion in 1 tablespoon olive oil. Pair with 1 small slice cantaloupe.

5. On-the-go nut butter toast: Spread 2 tablespoons almond or peanut butter on 1 slice toasted reduced-carb bread.

Try Tofu in the Morning!

Instead of eggs, cube and cook 4 to 6 ounces of silken tofu with chopped onion in 1 tablespoon olive oil. Sprinkle with a little curry powder while cooking, for flavor and visual appeal. Top with $1/4$ cup low-fat cheese. Pair with $1/2$ cup watermelon or add veggies of your choice to your tofu scramble.

Lunch

1. Classic tuna melt: Drain 1 small can light tuna and mix with 1 tablespoon olive oil mayonnaise. Heap onto 1 slice low-carb bread and top with 1 slice cheese. Melt the cheese in a toaster oven or carefully in your broiler. Enjoy with a tossed green salad and 1 tablespoon of your favorite dressing.

2. Steak salad: Top 4 cups of greens with 3 ounces sliced grilled or broiled steak, scallions, $1/4$ cup chopped red peppers, and $1/4$ cup mushrooms. Drizzle with 1 tablespoon oil-and-vinegar dressing. Pair with a slice of low-carb bread.

3. Fancy chicken and greens: Top 4 cups salad greens with 4 to 6 ounces sliced cooked chicken, $1/2$ cup sliced cucumber, 19 pecan halves, $1/4$ cup crumbled blue cheese, and a sprinkling of oil and vinegar. Pair with $1/2$ slice low-carb bread or a small slice of melon.

4. Chicken wrap sandwich: Spread a low-carb tortilla with 1 tablespoon olive-oil mayonnaise, then layer on 4 to 6 ounces sliced chicken, $1/2$ sliced avocado, $1/4$ cup shredded low-fat cheese, and fresh cilantro leaves. Roll and enjoy. Pair with $1/3$ cup watermelon.

5. Turkey pesto sandwich: Cut 1 slice low-carb bread in half or use a low-carb tortilla. To make your sandwich, fill with 3 ounces sliced turkey breast, lettuce leaves, roasted red pepper slices, and this pesto mix: 1 tablespoon mayonnaise combined with 1 teaspoon (or more to taste) fresh or dried chopped basil, a sprinkle of Parmesan cheese, and 1 tablespoon chopped walnuts (garlic lovers—add a shake of garlic powder or pressed juice from 1 small clove of garlic).

Dinner

1. Veggie burger 'n' "fries": Enjoy a Boca burger or other veggie burger on 1 slice low-carb bread, topped with 1 slice low-fat cheese. Pair with jicama "fries"—1 cup sliced jicama tossed with 1 tablespoon olive oil and spices of your choice, then baked on a greased cookie sheet at 375°F for 15 minutes.

2. Steak dinner: Have 4 to 6 ounces grilled or broiled steak, topped with mushrooms and onions sautéed in 1 tablespoon olive oil. Pair with 1 cup steamed green beans topped with 2 tablespoons chopped walnuts and

2 teaspoons olive oil. Add a small green salad topped with 2 tablespoons oil-and-vinegar dressing.

3. Supermarket rotisserie chicken feast: Enjoy 4 to 6 ounces of rotisserie chicken paired with 3 cups mixed greens topped with 2 tablespoons chopped walnuts, and 1 cup steamed broccoli (buy presliced or from the salad bar). Sweet ending: $\frac{1}{2}$ cup watermelon or cantaloupe chunks.

4. Pick 'n' peel shrimp meal: Pair boiled or steamed shrimp (buy precooked or cook at home) with 1 cup easy low-carb coleslaw. Make the slaw with bagged, preshredded coleslaw vegetables from the supermarket produce department, mixed with this easy dressing: $\frac{1}{2}$ cup olive oil mayo, $\frac{1}{2}$ cup half-and-half, 2 to 3 tablespoons white or cider vinegar (to thin the mixture to the consistency of a medium-thick dressing), celery seed and black pepper to taste, and $\frac{1}{2}$ packet or more of stevia for sweetness. Enjoy with a small green salad and $\frac{1}{2}$ cup watermelon cubes.

5. Easy leftovers stir-fry: Cook 4 to 6 ounces sliced chicken, beef, or lean pork or cubed tofu with $\frac{1}{4}$ cup chopped onions, 1 cup mushrooms, and $\frac{1}{2}$ cup sliced carrots (add garlic if desired) in 1 tablespoon olive oil. Serve over shirataki noodles. Pair with a green salad and 1 tablespoon dressing of your choice.

5 Snacks/5 Grams

These filling snacks have just 5 grams of carbs apiece and fit with ease into low-carb days on the 2-Day Diet.

1. Ham-and-cheese rolls: Slice a low-fat mozzarella stick in half lengthwise. Roll a slice of reduced-sodium deli ham around each stick. For crunch, add lettuce leaves or cucumber slices before rolling up.

2. Eggs and nuts: Have 2 hard-cooked eggs and a small handful of your favorite nuts.

3. Celery with peanut butter: Enjoy 2 to 3 celery sticks with 2 tablespoons creamy or crunchy peanut butter.

4. Cukes and hummus: Pair $\frac{1}{2}$ cup sliced cucumber with 3 tablespoons hummus.

5. Tomato and mozzarella: Top slices of fresh tomato with 2 ounces sliced part-skim mozzarella. Nice touch: Add fresh basil.

Mix-and-Match Meals

Looking for the easiest way to eat on the 2-Day Diet? Just follow our supersimple mix-and-match chart for low-carb and regular-carb days. Choose one food from each column and you'll have a healthy meal in minutes! Our test panelists loved this option, which helped them make great food choices on their busiest days. It's also an easy way to create low-carb lunches and dinners without following a recipe. Follow these rules:

CHOOSE YOUR PROTEIN	ADD A FLAVORFUL FAT
◆ 1 small can of light tuna	◆ 1 Tbsp olive or canola oil
◆ 4–6 oz canned chicken	◆ 1 Tbsp coconut oil
◆ 4–6 oz canned salmon	◆ 1 oz grated or sliced cheese
◆ 4 oz skinless chicken breast or turkey breast	◆ 2 Tbsp whole or chopped nuts
◆ 4 oz lean beef, burger, ground meat, or lean pork	◆ ¼ cup sliced, cubed, or mashed avocado
◆ 4–6 oz fish	Use your fats to cook with and to dress up your vegetables.
◆ 2 oz cheese (regular or reduced-fat)	
◆ 1 cup tofu	
◆ 2 eggs	
◆ 2 Tbsp peanut butter or almond butter	

Have a snack! On low-carb days, stick to snacks suggested in the diet plan or choose a high-protein snack such as natural cold cuts rolled up in lettuce or spinach leaves with a dab of mustard or mayo. Or try 2 tablespoons of peanut butter or almond butter on 1 celery stalk.

EASY LOW-CARB EATING

- Stick to about 50 total grams of carbs for the day.
- Aim for about 15 grams of carbs per meal plus about 5 grams in your daily snack.
- Eating out? Choose a meal similar to one in the plan—like a salad with cheese, chicken, and dressing; or a stir-fry with beef (or another protein) and a low-carb veggie like greens or scallions.
- Hungry? Have a little more protein with your meals.

FILL THREE-FOURTHS OF YOUR PLATE WITH VEGETABLES	FIT IN A LITTLE LOWER-CARB FRUIT
- On low-carb days, skip starchy, higher-carb veggies such as corn, lima beans, and potatoes. - Enjoy plenty of salad greens and cooked leafy greens. - Mixed green salads, baby spinach, red leaf lettuce, and radicchio are all low in carbs, as are cooked leafy greens such as spinach, kale, collards, mustard greens, and Swiss chard. Enjoy as much of these as you like. - Add ½ cup of another nonstarchy veggie, cooked or raw.	- ½ cup cubed casaba melon: 5.5 g carbs - ½ cup diced watermelon: 5.5 g carbs - ½ cup sliced strawberries: 6.5 g carbs - ½ cup diced cantaloupe: 6.5 g carbs - 1 medium plum: 7 g carbs - ½ cup blackberries: 7 g carbs - ½ cup raspberries: 7.5 g carbs - ½ medium grapefruit: 10.5 g carbs

Make it easy: Buy boxes and bags of prewashed salad greens and spinach (also in microwavable bags).
Make it fast: Look for precut vegetables like presliced carrots and broccoli; use bagged coleslaw mix (no dressing) as a mixed-vegetable dish.
No-waste options: Keep plain frozen vegetables on hand. Canned vegetables are good, too. (Use reduced-sodium varieties.)

GET CREATIVE!

Have a hankering for a favorite dish that's not on our meal plan or in our recipe section? Turn to "Create Your Own Meals" in Appendix A, on page 275. It's a handy chart listing hundreds of foods, arranged by food group and including all the information you need—from calories and carbs to fiber and protein—to help you create a healthy, delicious, on-plan meal.

FAST FOOD ON THE 2-DAY DIET

Yes, you *can* hit the drive-thru or sit down to a quick, fast-food lunch or dinner on the 2-Day Diet. Here's how you can take advantage of healthier fast-food menu options and smaller portion sizes to stay on track on low-carb days *and* on regular-carb days—and even fit in a couple of treats like burgers, onion rings, and a little ice cream!

We've chosen options at eight of the largest fast-food chains that at press time met basic meal requirements for both types of days. Low-carb recommendations have about 15 grams of carbohydrates per meal; regular-carb options have about 450 calories per meal. When possible, we calculated *net carbs* by subtracting grams of fiber from total carbs to give a true picture of a food's impact on blood sugar.

We've read through the nutrition facts for thousands of menu items to find the healthiest meals—those that are lower in saturated fat and higher in produce and that, where possible, also provide a serving of calcium- and vitamin D–rich dairy.

First, some general guidelines. On low-carb and regular-carb days, order meats–such as chicken in salads and sandwiches—grilled, not crispy. You'll side-step breading and frying that adds dozens of grams of carbohydrates, hundreds of calories, and gobs of fat. Skip add-ons like croutons for salads, too. On regular-carb days, order sandwiches without butter, mayo, or other greasy dressings. And on all days, quench your thirst with zero-carb, zero-calorie sips of water, diet soda, unsweetened iced tea, coffee, or hot tea. Use the no-calorie, natural sugar alternative stevia to add sweetness to tea or coffee.

Arby's

Best Low-Carb Choice

#1: Salad with turkey and a zero-carb drink. Choose the Chopped Farmhouse Salad with Roast Turkey (7 net carbs), topped with one of these dressings:

Light Italian (3 carbs), Balsamic Vinaigrette (5 carbs), or Buttermilk Ranch (2 carbs). Sip a zero-carb drink.

Best Regular-Carb Choices

#1: Roast beef sandwich, fries, and a soda. Choose the Jr. Roast Beef (210 calories) and value-size Curly Fries (240 calories). Sip a diet soda or other zero-calorie drink.

#2: Hot ham-and-cheese sandwich, fries, and a soda. Have the Jr. Ham and Cheddar Sandwich (210 calories) and the value-size Curly Fries (240 calories). Sip a diet soda or other zero-calorie drink.

#3: Chicken sandwich, salad, and a drink. Choose the Jr. Chicken Sandwich (320 calories). Pair with a Chopped Side Salad with Light Italian Dressing (100 calories) and a zero-calorie drink.

Burger King

Best Low-Carb Choices

#1: Meal-size salad plus a zero-carb drink. Go for the "Tendergrill" Chicken BLT Garden Fresh Salad with dressing (10 net carbs), paired with water, unsweetened iced tea, diet soda, coffee, or hot tea. Best dressings: Ken's Citrus Caesar Dressing (4 carbs for the whole packet) or Ken's Ranch Dressing (2 carbs per packet).

#2: Chicken nuggets plus a salad and a zero-carb drink. Go for the 4-piece nuggets (13 grams carbs) and you'll have room for a Garden Side Salad with Ranch Dressing (4 net carbs) and a zero-carb drink.

Best Regular-Carb Choices

#1: Grilled chicken sandwich and a fat-free milk. Choose the "Tendergrill" Chicken Sandwich without mayo (400 calories), plus a fat-free milk (90 calories). Adding a Side Salad (25 calories) with one-third of a packet of Ken's Lite Honey Balsamic Dressing (120 calories) boosts your meal total to 498 calories, but you get a worthwhile serving of produce.

#2: Burger, onion rings, and a zero-calorie soda. Looking for classic fast food? Choose a Whopper Jr. without mayo or cheese (260 calories) or a regular Hamburger (240 calories) or regular Cheeseburger (280 calories), paired with value-size Onion Rings (150 calories) and a zero-calorie diet soda (or unsweetened tea, water, coffee, or hot tea).

#3: Salad and a fat-free milk. Choose the Garden Fresh "Tendergrill" Chicken Garden Salad (240 calories), paired with a half packet of Lite Honey Balsamic Dressing (60 calories) and a fat-free milk (90 calories).

#4: Veggie burger, salad, and tea or milk. Go vegetarian with the Veggie Burger without mayo (320 calories), a Side Salad (25 calories) with one-third of a packet of Lite Honey Balsamic Dressing (23 calories), and unsweetened tea (0 calories) or fat-free milk (90 calories).

Chick-fil-A

Best Low-Carb Choices

#1: Chicken sandwich and a drink. Order the Chargrilled Chicken Sandwich "protein style"—with tomato, wrapped in lettuce (5 carbs), plus Honey Roasted BBQ Sauce (2 carbs) or the 1 packet Buffalo Sauce (1 carb). Or have the regular Chicken Sandwich "protein style" (12 carbs), with one of the sauces recommended here. Sip a zero-carb drink.

#2: Chicken club sandwich and a drink. Have the Chargrilled Chicken Club Sandwich (chicken, provolone cheese, bacon) "protein style"—with tomato, wrapped in lettuce (5 carbs). Add Honey Roasted BBQ sauce (2 carbs) and a zero-carb drink.

#3: Chicken salad and a drink. Order the Chargrilled Chicken Garden Salad (11 carbs), top with 1 packet Blue Cheese Dressing (3 carbs). Add a zero-carb drink.

Best Regular-Carb Choices

#1: Chicken sandwich and a salad. Order the Chargrilled Chicken Sandwich (290 calories) or a regular Chicken Sandwich without butter (410 calories), along with a Side Salad (70 calories) with Light Italian Dressing (25 calories) and bottled water or other zero-calorie drink.

#2: Chicken wrap and fruit salad. Have the Chargrilled Chicken Cool Wrap (410 calories), the Fruit Cup (70 calories), and unsweetened tea or other zero-calorie drink.

#3: Salad, soup, and lemonade. Order the Chargrilled Chicken Garden Salad (180 calories), a medium Hearty Breast of Chicken Soup (120 calories), and a medium-size diet lemonade (20 calories).

#4: Nuggets and soup. Have the 8-Count Nuggets (260 calories), a medium Hearty Breast of Chicken Soup (120 calories), and a hot tea, coffee, or other zero-calorie drink.

Dairy Queen
Best Low-Carb Choice

#1: Chicken salad and a drink. Order a Grilled Chicken Salad (9 net carbs) with Fat-Free Ranch Dressing (5 carbs) or Fat-Free Italian Dressing (4 carbs) and a zero-carb drink.

Best Regular-Carb Choice

#1: Chicken wrap, salad, ice-cream cone, and a drink. Order a Grilled Chicken Wrap (280 calories), a Side Salad (20 calories) with Fat-Free Italian Dressing (15 calories), and a kid-size cone (170 calories vanilla, 180 calories chocolate). Sip a zero-calorie drink.

McDonald's
Best Low-Carb Choices

#1: A meal-size salad and a zero-carb drink. Pair salads with these healthier dressings (which are also low in saturated fat and calories): Newman's Own Low-Fat Balsamic Vinaigrette (3 carbs) or Newman's Own Low-Fat Family Recipe Italian Dressing (7 carbs). Great choices include:

- Premium Bacon Ranch Salad with Grilled Chicken (6 net carbs)
- Premium Caesar Salad with Grilled Chicken (6 net carbs)
- Premium Southwest Salad with Grilled Chicken (2 net carbs)

#2: 4-piece McNuggets, a side salad, and water, unsweetened tea, or a diet drink. Need a little crunch? Order the 4-piece Chicken McNuggets (12 carbs) with a Side Salad (3 net carbs). Use the dressing choices suggested previously. Sip a zero-carb drink.

Best Regular-Carb Choices

#1: A burger. Go for a "regular" Hamburger (250 calories) or a Cheeseburger (300 calories), and you've got room for a Side Salad (20 calories plus dressing) and a carton of calcium-rich low-fat milk (100 calories). Or have your burger with the Snack Size Fruit and Walnuts (210 calories) and a zero-calorie drink.

#2: Meal-size salad plus milk. Enjoy one of the full-meal salads recommended under low-carb options, all of which clock in at under 300 calories. Pair with a low-fat milk.

Subway

Best Low-Carb Choice

#1: Salad and a drink. Choose any salad (except Sweet Onion Chicken Teriyaki) from the "Salads with 6 grams of fat or less" menu. These include Black Forest Ham, Oven Roasted Chicken, Roast Beef, Turkey Breast, and Veggie Delite. Each has 9 to 12 carbs. Top with one of these dressings: Oil and Vinegar (0 carbs), Chipotle Southwest (2 carbs), or Ranch (3 carbs). Sip a zero-carb drink.

Best Regular-Carb Choices

#1: Soup, salad, and a drink. Choose any salad from the "Salads with 6 grams of fat or less" menu (calories range from 50 for the Veggie Delite to 200 for the Sweet Onion Chicken Teriyaki). Top with one of these dressings: Fat Free Italian (35 calories) or Honey Mustard (80 calories). Add one of these soups: Minestrone (110 calories) or Tomato Garden Vegetable with Rotini (90 calories), Chicken Noodle or Spanish Style Chicken & Rice with Pork (110 calories each), or Chipotle Chicken Corn Chowder (130 calories). Sip a zero-calorie drink.

#2: Sandwich, soup, and a drink. Choose any of these sandwiches from the "Sandwiches with 6 grams of fat or less" menu: Veggie Delite (230 calories), Turkey Breast or Turkey Breast & Black Forest Ham (280 calories), or Black Forest Ham (290 calories). Pair with one of these soups: Minestrone or Tomato Garden Vegetable with Rigatoni (90 calories each), Chicken Noodle or Spanish Style Chicken & Rice with Pork (110 calories each), or Chipotle Chicken Corn Chowder (130 calories). Sip a zero-calorie drink.

#3: Chili, salad, and a milk. Order Chili con Carne (280 calories) and a Veggie Delite Salad (50 calories) with Fat Free Italian Dressing (35 calories); split a 12-ounce serving of low-fat milk (80 calories for a half serving).

Taco Bell

Best Low-Carb Choices

#1: Soft taco, guacamole, and a drink. Choose a Fresco Chicken Soft Taco (16 net carbs), a side of guacamole (2 carbs—add it to your taco), and a zero-carb drink.

#2: Crunchy taco, black beans, and a drink. Choose a Fresco Crunchy Taco (10 net carbs), a side of black beans (7 net carbs), and a zero-carb drink.

Best Regular-Carb Choices

#1: Chalupa, beans, and a zero-calorie drink. Choose a Chalupa Supreme Chicken (340 calories) or Steak (340 calories). Add guacamole to your chalupa (35 calories) or one or more of your favorite sauces at just 10 calories or less each: green tomatillo (10 calories); pico de gallo (5 calories); border sauce mild, hot, or fire; salsa (0 calories); or salsa verde (5 calories). Pair with a side of black beans (80 calories) and a zero-calorie drink.

#2: Burrito, beans, and a drink. Have a Fresco Bean Burrito (350 calories) or a Fresco Burrito Supreme Chicken or Steak (340 calories) with guacamole or one or more of the sauces recommended in #1. Add a side of black beans (80 calories) and a zero-calorie drink.

Wendy's

Best Low-Carb Choices

#1: Salad plus a zero-carb drink. Go for a half-size Apple Pecan Chicken Salad (11.5 net carbs), a full-size Chicken BLT Cobb Salad (6 net carbs), or a half-size Spicy Chicken Caesar Salad (12 net carbs), topped with one of these dressings: Avocado Ranch (2 carbs), Lemon Garlic Caesar (2 carbs), Light Classic Ranch (2 carbs), or Italian Vinaigrette (4 carbs). Pair with a zero-carb drink.

#2: Burger or grilled chicken on a lettuce "bun" with a side salad and a zero-carb drink. We love this! Order a quarter-pound hamburger patty (0 carbs) or the Ultimate Chicken Grill (3 carbs) on lettuce (1–2 carbs) instead of a regular bun. Pair with a Caesar or Garden Side Salad (3 net carbs) and one of the dressings recommended in #1. Sip a zero-carb drink.

#3: Chicken nuggets, salad, and a zero-carb drink. Go for the 4-piece Chicken Nuggets (10 net carbs); skip dipping sauces, which add 3 to 11 carbs. Pair with a Caesar or Garden Side Salad (3 net carbs) and a half-packet of Avocado Ranch, Lemon Garlic Caesar, or Light Classic Ranch (all are 1 carb for a half-packet). Sip a zero-carb drink.

Best Regular-Carb Choices

#1: Burger, fries, and a diet soda. Go for the Jr. Hamburger (250 calories), share some of your Value Natural-Cut Fries (whole serving is 230 calories), and sip a diet soda or other zero-calorie drink.

#2: Chicken sandwich and a salad. Order the Ultimate Chicken Grill (400 calories) with a Garden Side Salad (25 calories), topped with a half-packet of Light Classic Ranch (25 calories for the half-packet). Sip a zero-calorie drink.

#3: Meal-size salad plus a milk. We like the BLT Cobb Salad (390 calories) with a half-packet of Light Classic Ranch Dressing (25 calories for the half-packet). Sip a low-fat milk (100 calories)—it brings your meal total to 515, but you get a full serving of bone-friendly calcium.

#4: Chili, salad, and milk. Order the Large Chili (310 calories) and a Garden Side Salad (25 calories), topped with one-third of a packet of Light Classic Ranch (12 calories for one-third of a packet). Sip a low-fat milk (100 calories).

Fast-Food Breakfast Tips

Grabbing a quick morning meal? Find one that's closest to the recommended 2-Day Diet guidelines—15 grams of carbs on low-carb days, 450 calories on regular-carb days—by using these strategies:

Low-Carb Breakfast Options: Eggs, egg whites, or egg substitute cooked any style. Breakfast meats such as bacon, ham, or sausage. Omelet or scrambled eggs with onions, mushrooms, or spinach.

Low-Calorie Breakfast Options: Fruit salad. Two scrambled eggs. A small (2-egg) omelet with vegetables. Oatmeal with fruit and low-fat or fat-free milk. English muffin or toast and peanut butter. Yogurt with fresh fruit.

CASUAL DINING ON THE 2-DAY DIET

Yes, you *can* go out to lunch or dinner on the 2-Day Diet. As our test panelists discovered, eating out's a breeze on this plan. Many found that by sticking with favorite choices such as grilled chicken and salad, they could enjoy a meal out without overdoing carbs on low-carb days or without overeating on regular-carb days.

But what if you're not in the mood for a simple salad? We checked the nutrition information provided by 12 of America's largest casual-dining chain restaurants for more options. We were impressed by the wide range of delicious and inventive choices, and you will be, too. Just remember to choose a zero-carb, zero-calorie drink with your meal—sip some water, unsweetened iced tea, diet soda, hot tea, or coffee. You're all set for a great meal out!

Applebee's

Best Low-Carb Choices

#1: Steak and veggies. Order the 7-ounce House Sirloin (0 carbs) with two sides of seasonal vegetables (3–9 net carbs per serving).

#2: Chicken or steak Caesar salad. Order the regular-size Chicken Caesar Salad (16 net carbs) or Steak Caesar Salad (17 net carbs) without dressing. Top with Blue Cheese or Buttermilk Ranch Dressing (less than 1 carb per serving).

#3: Grilled shrimp salad with a side of veggies. Order the regular-size Grilled Shrimp 'N Spinach Salad (10 net carbs). Top with Blue Cheese or Buttermilk Ranch Dressing (less than 1 carb per serving). Add a side of another vegetable (3–9 net carbs).

Best Regular-Carb Choices

#1: Options from the lower-calorie menu. Applebee's offers several full meals under 550 calories on the chain's "Unbelievably Great Tasting & Under 550 Calories" menu. Options, which come with side dishes, include Roasted Garlic Sirloin (450 calories), Roasted Garlic Sirloin, and Napa Chicken & Portobellos (at 450 calories for the entrée with side dishes).

#2: Steak and potatoes. Order the 7-ounce House Sirloin (250 calories) with a seasonal vegetable (35–60 calories) and an order of Fried Red Potatoes (150 calories).

#3: Salad. Order the regular-size Grilled Chicken Caesar Salad without dressing (370 calories). Top with one-half of a serving of Mexi-Ranch Dressing (45 calories).

#4: Soup and salad. Order a bowl of Chicken Tortilla Soup (200 calories) or Chicken Noodle Soup (120 calories). Pair with Applebee's House Salad without dressing (120 calories), topped with one-fourth of a serving of Mexi-Ranch Dressing (45 calories).

Boston Market
Best Low-Carb Choices

#1: Rotisserie chicken plus sides. Choose one-quarter of a Rotisserie Chicken—white meat, no skin (1 carb)—or Rotisserie Chicken Three-Piece Dark Meat, skinless (1 carb). Pair with Green Beans (9 carbs), Fresh Steamed Vegetables (8 carbs), or Broccoli with Garlic Butter (6 carbs). Split a Caesar Salad (without croutons or chicken) with Oil and Vinegar Dressing (half of the salad with dressing is 4 carbs).

#2: Turkey and sides. Choose regular or large Turkey Breast (0 carb). Pair with Green Beans (9 carbs), Fresh Steamed Vegetables (8 carbs), or Broccoli with Garlic Butter (6 carbs). Split a Caesar Salad (without croutons or chicken) with Oil and Vinegar Dressing (half of the salad with dressing is 4 carbs).

Regular-Carb Choices

#1: Chicken, potatoes, and veggies. Order the 3-piece Dark Rotisserie Chicken (thigh and 2 drumsticks, no skin—280 calories) or one-quarter White Rotisserie Chicken (no skin—220 calories). Pair with Garlic Dill New Potatoes (100 calories) and Fresh Steamed Vegetables (80 calories).

#2: Beef, veggies, and cornbread. Order Beef Brisket (4 ounces—230 calories), Fresh Steamed Vegetables (80 calories), and Cornbread (160 calories).

#3: Chicken sandwich and salad. Order Half Rotisserie Chicken Carver Sandwich (340 calories) and Garlic Dill New Potatoes (100 calories).

Carrabba's Italian Grill
Best Low-Carb Choices

#1: Shrimp scampi. Order the Shrimp Scampi without the bread (9 carbs). Pair with Asparagi Alla Romano (3 carbs), Cauliflower Arrosto (5 carbs), or Sautéed Broccoli and Cauliflower (6 net carbs).

#2: Chicken, steak, or seafood salad. Choose Caesar Salad with Chicken (16 net carbs), Italian Cobb Salad with Sirloin (14 net carbs), or Italian Cobb Salad with Salmon or Shrimp (13 net carbs). Carb totals include Light Balsamic Vinaigrette Dressing.

#3: Chicken, pork, sirloin, or veal marsala. A full order of any of these has just 3 to 8 carbs. Pair with Asparagi Alla Romano (3 carbs), Cauliflower Arrosto (5 carbs), or Sautéed Broccoli and Cauliflower (6 net carbs).

#4: Chicken Parmesan. Order a small portion of Chicken Parmesan (8 net carbs). Pair with one or two of the vegetable sides recommended in #3.

#5: Grilled chicken or fish fillet. Order Chicken Bryan (9 carbs), Filet Fiorentina (1 carb), Filet Marsala (3 carbs), Filet Scampi (8 carbs), Grilled Chicken (1 carb), or Grilled Salmon (2 carbs) from the Wood-Burning Grill section of the menu. Pair with sides recommended in #3.

Best Regular-Carb Choices

#1: Chicken as you like it. Order Grilled Chicken (287 calories), a small serving of Chicken Marsala (342 calories), or a small serving of Chicken Parmesan (313 calories). Pair with Sautéed Spinach (35 calories) and either Grilled Vegetables (92 calories) or Primavera Arrosto (70 calories).

#2: Pasta. Order Spaghetti Pomodoro with whole grain spaghetti (431 calories). Pair with Sautéed Spinach (34 calories).

#3: Soup and salad. Order a bowl of Minestrone (235 calories) or Sicilian Chicken Soup (242 calories). Pair with a side-order-size Italian Salad with Light Balsamic Vinaigrette (100 calories).

Cheesecake Factory
Best Low-Carb Choices

#1: A smaller-size salad. Choose a BLT Salad (15 carbs); Boston House Salad (11 carbs); Endive, Pecan & Blue Cheese Salad (16 carbs); or the lunch-size Caesar Salad (9 carbs).

#2: Tuna or salmon with vegetables. Order Grilled Tuna (3 carbs) or Herb-Crusted Filet of Salmon (8 carbs). Pair with the Boston House Salad (10 carbs) or with Broccoli (9 carbs), Green Beans or Spinach (6 carbs each).

#1: Try the Weight-Management Grilled Chicken (580 calories), Grilled Mahi (470 calories), Seared Tuna Takati Salad (440 calories), or Weight-Management Salads (510–570 calories).

Chipotle Mexican Grill

Best Low-Carb Choices

#1: Burrito bowl. Create your own dish by choosing items as you walk along a cafeteria-style line. Make it low-carb with one of these combinations.

- A double portion of fajita vegetables (6 net carbs), chicken (1 carb), cheese (0 carbs), guacamole (2 net carbs)

- Black or pinto beans (12 net carbs), carnitas (seasoned pork—1 carb), cheese (0 carbs)

- Fajita vegetables (3 net carbs), steak (0 carbs) or barbacoa (seasoned beef—2 carbs), cheese (2 carbs), fresh tomato salsa (4 carbs)

- Fajita vegetables (3 net carbs), black beans (12 net carbs), green tomatillo salsa (2 net carbs)

#2: Salad with chicken, steak, carnitas, or barbacoa. Choose lettuce (2 carbs) topped with chicken (1 carb), steak (2 carbs), carnitas (1 carb), or barbacoa (2 carbs), plus a double portion of fajita vegetables (6 net carbs), cheese (0 carbs), and guacamole (2 net carbs).

Best Regular-Carb Choices

#1: Chicken and beans burrito bowl. Choose chicken (190 calories), black beans (120 calories), fajita vegetables (20 calories), and corn salsa (80 calories).

#2: Steak and guacamole burrito bowl. Choose steak (190 calories), pinto beans (120 calories), guacamole (150 calories), and fajita vegetables (20 calories).

#3: Beans, rice, and vegetable burrito bowl. Choose fajita vegetables (20 calories), pinto beans (120 calories), brown rice (160 calories), and guacamole (150 calories).

#4: Carnitas and vegetables. Choose a double portion of fajita vegetables (40 calories), carnitas (190 calories), brown rice (160 calories), and roasted chili-corn salsa (80 calories).

Olive Garden

Best Low-Carb Choices

#1: Salmon. Order Herb-Grilled Salmon (3 net carbs). Pair with a serving of Garden-Fresh Salad (9 net carbs with dressing).

#2: Chicken and greens. Have the Grilled Chicken Caesar Salad (14 net carbs).

#3: Soup and salad. Have a serving of Pasta e Fagioli (11 net carbs), plus a serving of salad (9 net carbs).

Best Regular-Carb Choices

#1: A fancy chicken dish. Order Venetian Apricot Chicken (400 calories for a dinner portion, 290 calories for a lunch portion). Enjoy with a serving of Garden-Fresh Salad without dressing (60 calories).

#2: Salad and soup. Enjoy a serving of Garden-Fresh Salad with dressing (150 calories). Pair with a serving of Pasta e Fagioli (130 calories), Minestrone (100 calories), or Zuppa Toscana (170 calories) and one breadstick with garlic-butter spread (140 calories).

Outback Steakhouse

Best Low-Carb Choices

#1: Steak and veggies. Choose the 6-ounce Outback Special Steak or the 6-ounce Victoria's Filet (0 carbs each). Pair with two or three of these sides: Grilled Asparagus (1 net carb), Seasonal Mixed Veggies (5 net carbs), Steamed Broccoli (5 net carbs), or Steamed Green Beans (1 net carb).

#2: Salmon dinner. Choose Norwegian Salmon (2 carbs) and two or three of the recommended sides in #1.

#3: Chicken and sides. Choose Alice Springs Chicken (13 carbs) or Grilled Chicken on the Barbie (10 carbs), plus Steamed Green Beans (1 net carb) and Grilled Asparagus (1 net carb).

Best Regular-Carb Choices

#1: Chicken night out. Choose Grilled Chicken on the Barbie (305 calories), Steamed French Green Beans (55 calories), and Grilled Asparagus (52 calories).

#2: Pork chops and sides. Order the Wood-Fire Grilled Pork Chop (383 calories) with Steamed Broccoli (109 calories).

#3: Steak and mashed potatoes. Order Victoria's Filet (6 ounces—218 calories). Share an order of Garlic Mashed Potatoes (152 calories for half an order) and Steamed French Green Beans (55 calories).

#4: Steak and salad. Pair Victoria's Filet (6 ounces—216 calories) with a House Salad with Tangy Tomato Dressing (215 calories).

P.F. Chang's China Bistro
Best Low-Carb Choice

#1: Shrimp plus a side dish. Order Shanghai Shrimp with Garlic Sauce (9 net carbs) or Shrimp with Lobster Sauce (15 net carbs), with Spicy Green Beans or Spinach Stir-Fried with Garlic (4 net carbs each).

Best Regular-Carb Choices

#1: Soup, salad, and dumplings for lunch. Order a cup of Wonton Soup (50 calories), Egg Drop Soup (60 calories), or Hot and Sour Soup (70 calories). Pair with a lunch-size portion of the Mixed Green Salad with Ginger or Sesame Dressing (200 calories for salad and dressing) or with Lime Dressing (110 calories for salad and dressing), and Steamed Dumplings with Lemongrass Chicken (130 calories) or Shrimp (110 calories). (Skip the dumpling sauce.)

#2: Chicken with broccoli. Order the Ginger Chicken with Broccoli (470 calories without rice).

#3: Salad with chicken or tuna. Order the Seared Ahi Tuna Wasabi Salad with Lemon Wasabi Dressing (470 calories) or the Thai Basil Green Salad with Chicken and Ginger-Lime Vinaigrette (438 calories).

#4: Shrimp your way. Order Shrimp with Lobster Sauce (320 calories), Sichuan Shrimp (360 calories), or Shanghai Shrimp with Garlic Sauce (240 calories). Have with one-third of an order of brown rice (103 calories).

#5: Lots of veggies. Order Buddha's Feast Steamed Veggies (260 calories), paired with half an order of brown rice (155 calories). Or have Buddha's Feast Stir-Fried Veggies (420 calories without rice).

Red Lobster

Note: This chain restaurant's focus on seafood and use of several low-carb/low-calorie cooking methods (broiling, grilling, steaming) means that many main dishes are both low-carb *and* lower in calories. You can order any of these on a low-carb or on a regular-carb day.

#1: Shrimp. Order the Shrimp Scampi (0 carbs, 130 calories), along with two of these sides: Fresh Asparagus (5 carbs, 60 calories), Broccoli (6 carbs, 45 calories), Garden Salad (13 carbs, 90 calories), with a half-serving of Balsamic Vinaigrette Dressing (2 carbs, 40 calories, for a half-serving). On a regular-carb day, you could also choose one side plus a Cheddar Bay Biscuit (150 calories).

#2: Lobster. Choose Steamed Lobster (0 carbs, 230 calories). Enjoy a little butter on low-carb days; skip it on regular-carb days to save calories. Pair with two of the sides suggested in #1.

#3: Crab. Order 1 pound of Snow Crab Legs (0 carbs, 180 calories) with any two of the sides suggested in #1.

#4: Fresh fish. Order any fresh fish grilled, broiled, or blackened. Carb counts range from 6 for haddock and halibut, to 7 for mahi mahi, to 10 for cod, and 11 for flounder. Calories range from 240 for sole, 300 for perch, 350 for flounder, 360 for lake whitefish and mahi mahi, to 410 for rainbow trout and 490 for salmon. Pair with sides recommended in #1.

Red Robin

Best Low-Carb Choices

#1: Wrap burgers in lettuce. Instead of a bread bun, opt for a lettuce wrap and save dozens of carbs. Order the Lettuce-Wrapped Burger (7 carbs), the Lettuce-Wrapped Veggie Burger (8 net carbs), or the Lettuce-Wrapped Grilled Chicken (4 carbs). Pair with Steamed Broccoli (3 net carbs) and a side order of Caesar Salad (4 net carbs).

#2: Chicken salad. Choose the Simply Grilled Chicken Salad without croutons or bread (12 carbs).

Regular-Carb Choices

#1: Chicken wrap. Order a Caesar's Chicken Wrap without the Creamy Caesar dressing (489 calories).

#2: Soup and salad. Order 2 cups of Chicken Tortilla Soup (279 calories) with a Side House Salad with dressing (115 calories) and Freckled Fruit Salad (97 calories).

#3: Grilled chicken sandwich and sides. Order a Grilled Chicken Sandwich (409 calories on a bun, 159 calories in a lettuce wrap). Pair with a side of Broccoli (32 calories). Add Southwest Black Beans (98 calories) if you've opted for the lettuce wrap.

Ruby Tuesday

Best Low-Carb Choices

#1: Chicken as you like it. Choose Chicken Bella (3 net carbs) or Plain Grilled Chicken (0 carbs). Pair with two or three of these sides: Sugar Snap Peas (5 net carbs), Sautéed Baby Portabella Mushrooms (2 net carbs), Fresh Grilled Asparagus (2 net carbs), Fresh Grilled Green Beans (3 net carbs), Fresh Grilled Zucchini (3 net carbs), or Roasted Spaghetti Squash (4 net carbs).

#2: Grilled steak dinner. Choose Plain Grilled Petite Sirloin (5 carbs) or Plain Grilled Top Sirloin (3 carbs). Pair with two or three of the sides recommended in #1.

#3: Seafood supper. Order the Creole Catch (0 carbs), Fit & Trim Grilled Salmon (0 carbs), Herb-Crusted Tilapia (9 net carbs), or New Orleans Seafood (2 carbs). Pair with two or three of the sides recommended in #1.

Best Regular-Carb Choices

#1: Fit & Trim Menu options. Most entrées and sides fit the 2-Day Diet guidelines for regular-carb days. Great choices include Petite Sirloin (376 calories), Barbecue Grilled Chicken (345 calories), Grilled Salmon (483 calories), and Spaghetti Squash Marinara (260 calories). Pair with sides such as Sliced Tomatoes with Balsamic Vinaigrette (52 calories), Fresh Grilled Green Beans (45 calories), and Fresh Grilled Asparagus (78 calories).

#2: Seafood plus sides. Opt for Crab Cake Dinner (270 calories), Grilled Salmon (389 calories), Creole Catch (240 calories), Jumbo Skewered Shrimp (242 calories), Herb-Crusted Tilapia (401 calories), or New Orleans Seafood (365 calories). Add one of the sides recommended in #1.

T.G.I. Friday's

Best Low-Carb Choices

#1: Salmon and lobster. Order Grilled Salmon with Langostino Lobster (6 carbs). Pair with the Fresh Vegetable Medley (4 net carbs), Broccoli (5 net carbs), Ginger-Lime Slaw (5 carbs), or Tomato Mozzarella Salad (4 net carbs).

#2: Chicken salad. Order the Grilled Chicken Cobb Salad (7 net carbs) with one of these vinaigrette dressings: Avocado (3 carbs), Balsamic (7 carbs), Caesar (3 carbs), or Ranch (2 carbs).

#3: Steak and sides. Choose a 10-ounce Sirloin (2 carbs), a 10-ounce Sirloin with Grilled Shrimp Scampi (7 carbs), a 10-ounce Sirloin with Langostino Lobster (5 carbs), a 6-ounce Sirloin (2 carbs), or a Flat Iron Steak (2 carbs). Add two or three of the sides recommended in #1.

Best Regular-Carb Choices

#1: Steak and sides. Choose a 6-ounce Sirloin (370 calories) or a Flat Iron Steak (380 calories). Pair with Broccoli (50 calories) or Tomato-Mozzarella Salad (90 calories).

#2: Soup and salad. Choose the House Salad with Bread Stick (210 calories) and a half-serving of Low Fat Balsamic Vinaigrette (40 calories for a half-serving). Pair with Tortilla or Chicken Noodle Soup (250 calories each).

#3: Sandwich and a side. Order half of a California Club Sandwich (435 calories) plus a side of Broccoli (50 calories).

Kathy Rocchetti

AGE: 53

HEIGHT: 5'2"

POUNDS LOST: 3.4

INCHES LOST: 13.0, including 4.25 inches from her waist and 3 inches from her hips

HEALTH UPGRADE: Her blood pressure fell to a healthy level, and her LDL cholesterol dropped 6 points.

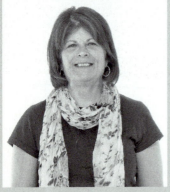

BEFORE

"My Shape Is Coming Back!"

Kathy Rocchetti's kitchen was a low-carb food festival during her 6 weeks on the 2-Day Diet—as she and her partner and their houseguests created endlessly varied stir-fries and paired grilled meats with vegetables and leafy salads.

"We did meat-and-vegetable kebabs and a lot of grilling with vegetables," says Kathy, an administrative assistant who's also going to college full-time to become a paralegal. "We even grilled radishes, which are very tasty. I asked everyone to go light on higher-carb vegetables like corn and peas."

All of them savored the creative salads that made their way onto the menu. "We always had a nice big salad and added new things all the time," she explains. "It wasn't just lettuce and tomatoes. We added fruit and nuts and lots of different vegetables." Kathy also auditioned several lower-carb substitutes for regular bread until she found a type she liked. "I tried lots of low-carb items like tapioca bread—that was definitely *not* a big hit—and low-carb wraps, which we all enjoyed."

As a result, Kathy lost pounds and a lot of inches. She's back in a pair of size 10 jeans that had been sidelined because they were too tight. "My waistline is more defined, my legs feel good, and my clothes fit better," she says. "My shape is coming back. I'm going to keep on going, to lose more weight."

She's just as thrilled by other changes. "My stomach had been bothering me—I felt bloated and uncomfortable before. I feel much better now that I'm eating fewer carbs," she says. "One day I had some spaghetti and didn't feel well afterward, so I'm trying to stay away from too many refined carbs."

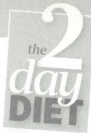

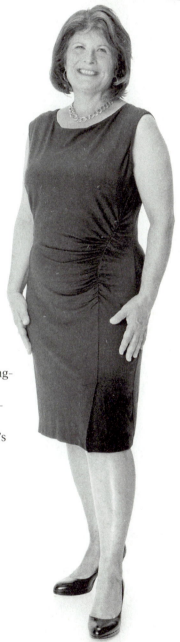

Sleep is easier now, too. "I fall asleep faster now and get right back to sleep if I wake up during the night," she says. "And I feel so much better in the morning. I used to have a lot of trouble falling asleep—I just couldn't get comfortable. I was shocked that changing my diet and getting more exercise could make such a difference. You don't think of food as the culprit behind so many issues. And I'm not as moody or hyper. I feel happy and not so stressed. I just feel good about myself."

At first, Kathy was worried that she'd feel hungry on the 2-Day Diet's 2 low-carb days each week. But she quickly realized that eating lean protein, vegetables, and smaller portions of higher-carb foods not only filled her up at meal-time, but kept her feeling satisfied longer. "Starches with a meal were just part of our upbringing in my family," she says. "Bread and potatoes were staples, and I always felt I was missing something if I didn't have a starch on the table. Now I know that you don't really have to have starch—it's okay to eat a second vegetable or a salad instead."

The plan's "no fail" approach meant small deviations never turned into big slides. "I went out for a special dinner one night and had a piece of strawberry-rhubarb pie—my ultimate favorite. It was delicious and I really enjoyed every single bite, but I got right back on track the next day," she says. "I was always careful about what I ate, but knowing that I had another chance coming up if I ate too many carbs on a low-carb day made it easier."

PART III

The 2-Day Diet work

Ready for our calorie-burning, fat-blasting, superefficient exercise program? Here's the workout plan at a glance:

DAY 1: PEAK INTERVAL WORKOUT PLUS ENDURANCE TONING ROUTINE

The 30-minute Peak Interval Workout alternates 15-second bursts of higher-intensity activity with longer, 45-second recovery periods. You'll blast fat and calories, lose pounds, and get energized!

The 15-minute Endurance Toning Routine uses light weights as you move through five multimuscle strength-training exercises. You'll burn more calories as you build muscle mass, which makes you look firmer, boosts metabolism so you burn more calories 24/7, and increases strength and endurance so everyday activities—from carrying groceries to dancing on Saturday night—are easier.

Total time investment: 45 minutes.

out

DAY 2: TEMPO INTERVAL WORKOUT PLUS POWER TONING ROUTINE

The 30-minute Tempo Interval Workout challenges you to sustain higher-intensity activity for 4 minutes, then recover during a minute of lower-intensity activity. By repeating this sequence, you'll boost stamina while losing weight.

The 15-minute Power Toning Routine uses heavier weights as you perform the same multimuscle strength-training moves that you did for the Endurance Toning Routine. Heavier weights and fewer repetitions build more sleek, sexy, strong muscle.

Total time investment: 45 minutes.

Ready to get started? Let's work it out!

CHAPTER 10

Prep for Exercise
Success

I t's easy! Follow a few simple rules and you'll get great results with the 2-Day Diet Workout. Here's what you need to know before you get started:

Rule #1: Do the workout twice a week. Each training session challenges your body in a unique way and delivers unique benefits, so you get a well-rounded exercise routine in just 90 minutes a week.

Use interval training while you walk or during any aerobic activity you enjoy, from biking to swimming to jogging. You can even do interval training in your living room: jumping rope or doing jumping jacks for the high-intensity bursts, marching or jogging in place for the lower-intensity recovery periods in between. Great for rainy days or when you want to catch your favorite TV show!

There are also two types of strength-training routines. Both use the same five exercises. But 1 day a week you'll use lighter weights and more repetitions to boost stamina with the Endurance Toning Routine. On the other day, you'll use heavier weights and lift them for fewer repetitions. This Power Toning Routine builds both strength and stamina.

Rule #2: Pick the days and times that work for you. Exercise at your convenience. And it's okay to do the strength and interval routines on separate days.

Rule #3: Follow the instructions! Let the interval training chart and strength-training directions and photos in Chapter 11 be your guide. Read the frequently asked questions ahead to find out more about adapting the program to meet your own needs and your schedule.

Rule #4: Warmup and cooldown. There's a 5-minute warmup built into the start of the interval-training workout. If you do the strength moves after that, your muscles will be sufficiently warm and flexible. If you do the strength moves alone, or do them first for more muscle building, spend a few minutes walking or even marching in place to warm up. Increasing the temperature of muscle tissue prevents injuries and makes exercise feel great, too.

And be sure to cool down after your interval workout. There's a cooldown built right into the routine. Don't be tempted to skip it to save time. It's important to decrease your heart rate and breathing rate gently and slowly, rather than transitioning abruptly from exercising to standing still.

Rule #5: Get your gear. Prep for success by making sure you have all the equipment you'll need. That includes walking shoes, socks, comfortable walking clothes, a water bottle, and some sort of timer for interval-training days. (Of course you'll also need the equipment for whatever aerobic activity you'll be doing with intervals, such as biking or swimming.) For strength-training routines, be sure to have two sets of dumbbells—a lighter set and a heavier set. Refer to page 231 for details on choosing the right weights for you.

WORKOUT Q&A

Our test panelists discovered that the 2-Day Diet Workout is as flexible as the eating plan. Here's what you need to know about fitting it in and adjusting it to meet your needs.

Q: I have knee pain. How can I adapt the strength-training moves to meet my needs?

A: Two of the five multipurpose strength-training moves in the 2-Day Diet Workout—the Plié Squat & Curl and the Lunge & Twist—involve bending your knees while you work out with weights. If you have knee pain, try the "Easier" advice for each exercise. These tips involve bending your knees less and keeping your feet on the floor, both of which take pressure off your knee joints. Don't bend your knees past 90 percent. Your knees should not extend past your toes.

If careful, easy bending isn't enough to keep you pain free, try standing up or sitting in a chair while doing just the upper-body parts of these moves.

The Kneeling Arm Raise, performed while you're on your hands and knees on the floor, can also be adapted. If kneeling bothers your knees, stand up, or do the arm moves while seated in a chair.

Of course, stop right away if your knees hurt or if you feel or hear clicking or grinding in your knee joints.

Q: *I have back problems and/or back pain. Can I do the 2-Day Diet strength-training moves?*

A: As with any health condition, it's smart to check in with your health care practitioner first. Everyone's pain is different. Let your doc see the photos of the strength-training moves and read the directions; discuss whether these moves are right for you and whether modifications can be made specifically for you.

Q: *I already have a regular exercise routine. Should I give it up for the 2-Day Diet Workout?*

A: No, just incorporate the principles behind the 2-Day Diet Workout into your regular routine. If you run, bike, hike, swim, walk more than 2 days a week, or love aerobic exercise classes, bring the superefficient concept of intervals into your routine. Two days a week, do intervals during your workout—or choose an exercise class that alternates faster-paced segments and slower-paced segments, as many do, to get the same effect. Interval training is more intense, so don't do it every day. Give yourself a rest day or two in between, when you go back to a more steady-paced routine.

If you're already strength training, keep it up! When you're pressed for time and would just like to give your muscles a new set of moves, try out the 2-Day Diet strength routine. Changing up your workout this way uses your muscles in new ways, which can improve your results.

Q: *I don't have 45 minutes to do the whole 2-Day Diet Workout. What can I do?*

A: Split it up. You could do the 30-minute interval routine one day and the strength routine another. You can even split up the interval workout into two 15-minute workouts on superbusy days. And it's okay to do one part of the strength routine at one time of day, the other part at another or even on a different day. Just be sure to leave at least 1 "rest day" between strength-training days so that your muscles can repair themselves and recover. (It's okay to do the interval routine on rest days.)

Q: *Some days I don't have time even for two 15-minute walks. Am I out of luck?*

A: Never! It's always better to do something than nothing. Break free of the all-or-nothing thinking that can keep you at your desk and use whatever pocket of time you have, even on a supercrazy day, for a brief interval walk.

You'll see benefits and probably feel them, too. Exercise can relax and energize you, restoring your mental focus on frantic days when you need it most.

Q: I walk with a friend and love the time we spend together. Having a walking buddy also ensures that we both get out there a couple of times a week. But when we do intervals, we walk at different speeds. What can we do so that we don't lose our social time?

A: Fitness expert Michele Stanten, who developed the 2-Day Diet Workout, suggests meeting at a local track, such as at the nearest high school or middle school, or at a loop trail, such as a local walking trail. Warm up together, then do intervals at your own pace. You'll still see and pass each other frequently. Walk together again for your cooldown. You may have to experiment to find the easiest way to meet up at the end. One of you may have to turn around and walk back to meet the other or cut across the middle of the track or loop, for example. But it's worth working out the details so that you can enjoy time together and still get in the best interval workout for each of you.

Q: Is it better to work out in the morning, the afternoon, or the evening?

A: Don't look to science to settle the debate about the best time of day to exercise. One informal survey of exercisers found that people who fit in their physical activity in the morning are more likely to stick with it—probably because the demands of the day don't derail your intentions as they can later on.[1] Then again, another study, from the Exercise Physiology Lab at the University of Louisville (Kentucky),[2] found that your muscles and joints are more flexible in midafternoon—probably because you've already been moving around for several hours, warming up your body. Body temperature is higher then, too. Still another study found that working out before breakfast seems to burn more fat than working out after your morning meal, though that strategy may leave you very hungry before your routine is done.[3]

The bottom line? Exercise at the time of day that works best for you. If you're not a morning person, find time during lunch or before or after dinner. The best exercise time slot is the one you can stick with.

Q: Should I stretch before or after the workout?

A: If you enjoy stretching, do it at the end of your routine. Your muscles will be warmed up already, and stretching moves will relax them and improve flexibility. Never stretch till it hurts—a stretch should feel good. (Some trainers, especially yoga instructors, suggest going for a "delicious" stretch, one that feels great.) Stretching can also help prevent stiffness and soreness in the 24 hours after your workout. Here are some stretches to try.

Bent-Leg Stretch. Stand and balance on your left leg. Hold on to a chair or countertop for support as you bend your right knee and grasp the top of your right foot with your right hand behind you, so that your right foot is up close to the back of your right thigh. Pull your heel upward toward your buttocks. Keep your right knee pointing down toward the ground. You'll feel a stretch in the front of your thigh. Hold for 10 seconds and release. Switch legs and repeat.

Lunge and Reach. Stand with your right foot positioned 2 to 3 feet in front of your left foot, toes pointed straight ahead. Bend your right knee slightly, and keep your left leg straight and the heel of your left foot on the floor. You'll feel a stretch in your calf and hip. You can hold on to a chair or countertop for support with your right hand. Reach up with your left arm, then reach slightly over your head toward the right so you also feel a stretch in your left side. Hold for 10 seconds and release. Switch legs and repeat.

Sit Back. Stand with your feet together, then with your left foot step back 6 to 12 inches. Straighten your right leg, lifting your front toes off the floor. Bend your left leg and sit back, placing your hands on your left thigh. It is very important not to lock your front knee. You should feel a stretch down the back of the thigh of your straight leg. Hold for 10 seconds and release. Switch legs and repeat.

Figure 4. Stand up. Put your right hand on your hip and use your left hand to hold on to a steady, sturdy support such as a chair or countertop for balance. Pick up your left foot and rest it on your right thigh, just above your right knee. Now "sit back" as if you were going to sit down—just enough to feel a stretch in your left hip and buttocks. Hold for 10 seconds and release. Switch legs and repeat.

Q: *Should I exercise if I'm sick?*

A: It all depends. The first rule is to pay attention to what your body is telling you. If you feel too sick for physical activity, take it easy. If you do work out, consider making it less intense. One way to decide whether or not to exercise is by doing a "neck check." In general, symptoms above your neck such as a runny nose or sore throat needn't stop you. In fact, a walk or other workout can energize you if you're feeling a little run-down.

But if your symptoms are below the neck, such as body aches, chills, an upset stomach, or diarrhea—or if they're bodywide, such as a fever—it's a good idea to take a break. Return to exercise when you feel better.

BE PREPARED!

Get ready today! A little prep will help you get the most from your interval-training and toning routines. These expert-designed routines are safe and effective. But be aware that lifting weights and exercising in higher-intensity bursts may not be right for you if you have a chronic medical condition or are more than 20 pounds overweight. Be sure to discuss the workout details with your doctor first if you have arthritis, asthma, diabetes, heart disease, high blood pressure, or osteoporosis (brittle bones). Ask about modifications to meet your specific needs, too.

What about gear? The good news is that you need just a few pieces of fitness "equipment" for the 2-Day Diet Workout. The basic list:

- Walking shoes

- Socks that wick moisture away from your skin

- A portable, easy-to-read timer to keep track of your intervals

- Comfortable walking clothing appropriate for outdoor walks, the gym, or your home treadmill

- Equipment for other cardio activity you'll be doing as your interval workout, such as a bathing suit and goggles, bike shorts, and shoes

- Two sets of dumbbells—a lighter set and a heavier set (read on to learn how to choose the right weight)

Gear Guide

Use these recommendations when shopping for gear and when checking what you already own.

Walking Shoes

You don't have to spend a fortune to get great walking shoes. In one study from the University of Dundee in Scotland, testers rated midpriced shoes as good as or better than expensive models for support, cushioning, and comfort.[4] Real

(continued on page 230)

Michelle Sparr

AGE: 29

HEIGHT: 5'1½"

POUNDS LOST: 3.2

INCHES LOST: 15, including 6 from her waist

HEALTH UPGRADE: Her blood pressure and triglycerides fell to healthier levels.

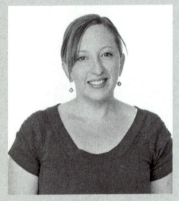

BEFORE

Afternoon Energy— Just in Time

Michelle Sparr is an on-call "computer doctor"—part of the team that keeps the electronics humming for hundreds of employees at a large publishing company. "In my job, there are lots of calls for help first thing in the morning and lots more right after lunch," she says. "I'm always busy. I move around all day, walking across parking lots and up and down stairs carrying equipment like monitors, desktop computers, laptops, and all kinds of accessories. I have to stay alert, solve problems, and stay positive while dealing with frustrated people whose computers aren't working."

But in the middle of her busy days, just when she needed a big energy boost, her lunches had been letting her down. She didn't realize that until she switched to lower-carb options on the 2-Day Diet. "I'd been eating only carbs for lunch and felt very tired and draggy in the afternoon," she says. "But after starting the program and having more protein and veggies, I have much more energy—without energy, I can't be productive."

When she started the 2-Day Diet, Michelle was getting ready to walk down the aisle as a bridesmaid in a close friend's wedding wearing a strapless, daffodil yellow dress made of smooth polished cotton. The dress was styled to fit snugly through the waist, then flared out into a cute short skirt. But it was a bit too snug. Would the dress fit on the big day? Just a few weeks into the program, Michelle had her last fitting—and found the dress was now loose and needed to be taken in nearly 2 inches. "That was definitely a bonus," she says.

A longtime yogurt fan, she made a big swap after reading the nutrition label on her usual

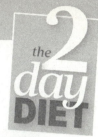

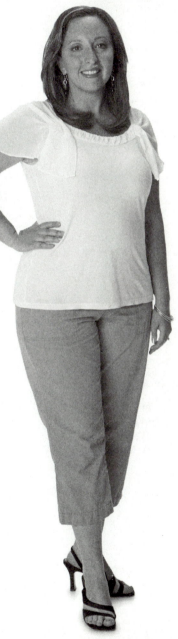

brand. "I was eating almost a day's worth of carbs in one yogurt," she says. "In the past, I'd only paid attention to calories and fat. But I still wanted to have yogurt, so I switched to plain nonfat Greek yogurt. I sweetened it with organic stevia and added strawberries, raspberries, or blueberries. It's great!"

She's ditched extra carbs in other places, too. Instead of having a bagel for breakfast, Michelle now chooses a slice of low-carb toast with peanut butter. Instead of a sandwich or pasta for lunch, it's a vegetable and protein or a sandwich on low-carb bread. "Then I'll have a balanced dinner—protein, vegetables, a little brown rice, or a second helping of the veggies."

Her biggest food challenges—being a picky eater and being a mom who cooks dinner every night for her husband and stepdaughter—were easy to overcome. "I don't eat eggs," she says. "So I stuck with the breakfast of yogurt, berries, and nuts from the 5-Day Jump Start. Since it was more protein than my usual breakfast, I stayed full longer in the morning."

She adapted several recipes to cook in her slow cooker, like the pork picadillo. "My family really liked it," she says. "I also don't eat seafood, so I used the mix-and-match meals chart to create other low-carb meals instead of meals with fish."

With the 2-Day Diet, Michelle revved up her afternoon slump—and kept her family healthy and happy at the same time. "I made a Chocolate-Almond Smoothie for my stepdaughter," Michelle says. "She really liked it."

walking shoes can help prevent injury, avoid pain, and stay comfy because they're built to support the heel-toe motion of walking. With a rounded or beveled heel and extra heel cushioning, a walking shoe helps you roll smoothly through your step, propelling you forward. (In contrast, running shoes have more cushioning at the midfoot because runners' feet strike the ground in a more flat-footed way. The heel may have less cushioning, too.)

It's smart to buy walking shoes in person rather than online, so you can try them on. Bring the socks you plan to wear while walking (read on for recommendations). Find a shoe store with a wide variety of walking shoes, such as a specialty walking-shoe store or athletic-shoe store. Shop in the late afternoon or evening, when your feet are biggest after carrying you through your day. But don't assume you know your shoe size. Ask to have your feet measured—aging, childbearing, and extra pounds can all lead to a larger foot size. Athletic shoes are sometimes sized a little differently from everyday shoes, so be ready to spend some time trying on larger and smaller sizes till you find the perfect fit.

Once you've narrowed down your shoe choices, put them through their paces. If the store has a treadmill, walk on it to see how your potential new shoes perform. If there's no treadmill, walk around the store or even outside (ask first, of course). The right shoe will feel good right out of the box, without a break-in period. Skip shoes that pinch, squeeze, rub, or slip at the heel.

Walking Socks

It's worth spending a few dollars on newer athletic socks made for walkers. These are made from wicking materials that keep your feet dry, comfortable, and blister-free. Sock materials worth checking out include CoolMax, Dri-Fit, and lightweight wools developed for active use such as Icebreaker and SmartWool. Newer socks may combine more than one of these materials for even better performance.

TEST PANELIST TIP: *Mash It!*

Instead of mashed potatoes, several test panelists tried—and fell in love with—mashed cauliflower. "It's so easy and delicious," says Anne Marie York. Panelist Nancy Barnes went a step further, mashing up other vegetables, including zucchini or tomatoes. "I'd try to have one regular vegetable and one mashed vegetable on my plate," she says, "so I didn't miss potatoes."

Be sure to check the sock size. Overly tight socks can cause blisters, while loose socks can bunch up. Special features found in "high performance" socks may help solve particular problems by providing extra padding in the heel and at the ball of the foot, odor control, and blister protection via special gels embedded in the material. Rumple-free, "anatomically correct" socks are designed to fit your left and right feet.

Timer

A watch with a second hand, or a sports watch or pedometer with a timer, can help you stay on track during your interval walks. Carrying one means you'll always know when it's time to start a fast-paced interval and when it's time to slow down.

Weights

Visit discount stores to find dumbbells for just a few dollars per set. You'll need lighter weights for endurance toning, plus a set of heavier weights for power toning. Shop when you'll have time to test various sizes.

To find light weights that are right for you, start with a pair of 1- or 2-pound dumbbells. Lift them 18 times (try a simple biceps curl). Can you keep going? If you can easily lift the weights more than 22 times, try a dumbbell that's 1 pound heavier. Ideally, you want a weight you can lift with good form no more than 18 to 20 times.

To find heavier weights, try out a pair of 5-pound dumbbells. Start lighter if that seems too heavy. Try to lift it 8 times. If you can do that, see if you can easily lift it more than 12 times. If you can, try a heavier weight. Aim for a weight that you can lift with good form 8 to 10 times but no more.

THE SECRETS OF WORKOUT SUCCESS

You've got your gear and you're ready to move. Following these strategies will help you get the most out of your routine.

Secret #1: Upgrade Your Walking Style

The secret to turning a stroll into a fat-blasting workout is using proper walking form and technique—especially when you pick up the pace during high-intensity bouts.

A common mistake people make when they walk faster is lengthening their stride. Did you know this can actually slow you down because your outstretched leg acts like a brake? It also puts more stress on your joints, boosting risk for injury.

A better idea: Take shorter, quicker steps, rolling from heel to toes and pushing off with your toes. Next, bend your arms at about 90-degree angles and swing them forward (no higher than chest height) and back so your hand is almost skimming your hip. Letting your arms flail across your body will slow down your forward momentum. Practice these techniques and you'll be cruising past other walkers in no time.

Secret #2: Use Good Form for Strength Training

Get the most out of your toning routine and reduce your risk for injury by following a few easy guidelines. First, read through the exercise descriptions and look at the photos before you start.

TEST PANELIST TIP: *Beyond Walking*

Nancy Barnes took her bike out for regular rides through the countryside while she was on the 2-Day Diet—and afterward. "I do 10 to 12 miles at a minimum," she says. "I live in an area with so many beautiful roads and bike trails. I love being outdoors!"

Paula Weiant joined a women's running program called First Strides. "You start out running for 1 minute and walking for 10 minutes, then gradually build up to running a 5-K [about 3 miles]," she says. "I'd been a walker for years and never lost weight, but running gave me a higher-intensity workout, and alternating between walking and running was a great interval routine."

During each exercise, be sure you keep breathing calmly. Don't hold your breath. Keep inhaling and exhaling to send energizing oxygen to every muscle cell in your body! Rest for a minute between exercises—longer if you're feeling tired. Don't rush. Do each move slowly and smoothly. And don't overexercise. One set of repetitions is enough to get results. Of course, if you feel pain during an exercise, stop immediately. Try it with a lighter weight the next time you work out.

Secret #3: Listen to Your Body

If you find the interval workouts or toning/strength routine so challenging that you're not sure you can finish, just do what you can. It's more important to exercise consistently than it is to push yourself so hard that you become overtired or achy or even risk injury. Work at your own pace, and when you feel at ease during your workout, try doing a little more. Over several weeks, aim to build your time, intensity, and/or number of weight repetitions. Test panelists who listened to their body this way got great results.

CHAPTER 11

The 2-Day Diet
workout

No matter what your goal is—to drop pounds, get healthy, feel younger, or reduce your risk of disease—exercise can help! And you don't have to be a gym rat to see the benefits. The 2-Day Diet exercise plan is designed to maximize results with just two 45-minute sessions a week. Each workout includes two main components:

- Cardio to build a healthier heart and lungs and burn lots of calories

- Toning to build muscle, make you stronger, and rev your metabolism

CARDIO: THE MAGIC OF INTERVAL TRAINING

The cardio workouts feature intervals. That means you'll be alternating between higher intensity (or harder bouts of exercise) and lower intensity (or easier bouts of exercise for recovery). This type of training has been shown to burn more calories and speed results compared with cardio workouts that are done at the same intensity from beginning to end. Each interval-training routine has two parts:

1. The Peak Interval Workout. You'll be doing supershort bouts—only 15 seconds—of vigorous exercise, with a longer recovery (45 seconds). The goal is to really push yourself. It's only 15 seconds, so you can do it, and it's worth the effort. This type of training will spike your calorie burn and challenge your body so you'll lose weight and get fit faster.

2. The Tempo Interval Workout. These are longer bouts—4 minutes peak and 1 minute recovery. Since you can't go all out for 4 minutes, you'll be working at a slightly lower (but still challenging) intensity, with less rest time. This type of training will boost your endurance and keep your calorie burn high.

TONING: BUILD SLEEK, METABOLISM-REVVING MUSCLE

Strength—or toning—workouts are essential to curb the decline in muscle mass, and the accompanying dip in metabolism, that occurs as you get older. By building more muscle, you'll keep your metabolism in high gear and you'll look toned and fit. You'll also be stronger, and the stronger you are, the easier everyday tasks become, so you can be more active throughout the day.

All the exercises in the 2-Day Diet Workout are combo moves, meaning they work multiple muscle groups at the same time for a more efficient workout that burns more calories than if you did exercises that isolate muscles.

On one day, you'll do the Endurance Toning Routine: You'll be doing more reps with lighter weights to boost your stamina.

On the other day, you'll do the Power Toning Routine: To crank up your strength gains, you'll use heavier weights and do fewer reps.

Just follow the instructions—and use the photos as your guide. It's fun and easy.

GETTING STARTED

In the pages ahead, you'll find directions and photos for this remarkable, time-saving workout plan. Take your time and read through this section completely before you begin. It may also be helpful to make copies of the directions, charts, and photos so that you can have them in front of you as you exercise.

TEST PANELIST TIP: *Go at Your Own Pace*

Michelle Sparr found that adding interval workouts to her walks felt hard at first. By listening to her body, she adjusted the routine to get a good workout without overdoing it. "I had to cut back sometimes on the number of intervals. I found I needed more recovery time between high-intensity intervals," she says. Remember: The goal isn't speed—*it's challenging your own body.*

Warm Up!

To prepare for your workouts, always perform a warmup to gradually increase your body temperature and increase blood flow to your exercising muscles. This will ease you into your workouts so you'll feel better and reduce your chances of an injury.

If you do the entire routine at the same time, you can change the order of the strength and cardio segments if you'd like. If your primary goal is to drop pounds, you should always do the cardio segment first. If your primary goal is to get toned, you should always do the strength segment first. If you want to achieve both, alternate the order each day.

Remember: If you do the cardio and strength routines at different times of the day or on separate days (that way, you'd end up exercising 4 days a week), always warm up before you begin either routine.

Know Your Intensity Level

Interval training is based on alternating bouts of higher-intensity and lower-intensity activity. How can you tell if you're working hard enough—and if you're giving yourself enough of a break during low-intensity recovery periods? We like to use a scale of 1 to 10, with 1 being lying on the couch and 10 being sprinting for your life.

Here's what various intensity levels feel like. Notice the four effort levels. You'll be seeing them throughout the 2-Day Diet Workout guide to interval training. Refer back to this chart if you're not sure what intensity you should be going for during a workout.

Exercise Intensity Levels—How They Feel

EFFORT LEVEL	INTENSITY LEVEL	HOW IT FEELS
A: Easy	3–4	Rhythmic breathing—you can sing.
B: Somewhat Hard	5–6	Breathing a bit harder—you can talk in complete sentences.
C: Hard	7–8	Slightly breathless—you can talk only in brief phrases.
D: Very Hard	9	Breathless—you don't want to talk, but you could manage yes/no answers.

DAY 1: PEAK INTERVAL WORKOUT PLUS ENDURANCE TONING ROUTINE

You can do this interval routine with your favorite cardio workout, from walking to jogging to taking on the elliptical machine. You could also do this in your living room: March or jog in place for the Level B intervals, and jump rope (or pretend to), do jumping jacks, or do other high-intensity moves for the Level D intervals.

The Warmup

Devoting a few minutes to warming up isn't a waste of time, so don't be tempted to skip it! Starting out slowly warms your muscles and makes joints and connective tissue more flexible—making movement easier and more enjoyable.

Day 1: Warmup

TIME (MINUTES)	WHAT TO DO
0:00–1:00	March or jog in place, swinging your arms at your sides. Walk or jog at an easy pace. If you're on a cardio machine, go at an easy pace. (If you're swimming, swim at an easy pace for 5 minutes.)
1:01–2:00	While doing your activity from the first minute, reach both arms overhead 20 times. Pump your arms at your sides for the remaining time.
2:01–3:00	Keep moving your legs and press your arms in front of you at chest height, then pull them back so your elbows are pointing behind you, hands by your chest. Do 20 times. Pump your arms at your sides for the remaining time.
3:01–4:00	Keep moving your legs and alternately circle each arm backward, palm facing away from you. Do 40 circles total, 20 with each arm. Pump your arms at your sides for the remaining time.
4:01–5:00	Return to marching or jogging in place, swinging your arms at your sides. Walk or jog at an easy pace. If you're on a cardio machine, go at an easy pace.

A longtime runner, Diane Mann added interval training to her 4-day-a-week routine—and suddenly, a half-hour run wasn't just a long slog.

"There's more variety with interval training," she says. "You're thinking about the seconds or minutes left in a fast or slow interval, so the time goes by so much faster. A steady-paced run is much more monotonous, but intervals make the same-length workout more effective and more fun."

Peak Interval Workout

Ready to burn calories, torch fat, and boost your fitness level? Peak intervals are a surprisingly doable way to add high-intensity training to your routine. You'll work at a faster pace for just 15 seconds at a time, then back off for 45 seconds to recover and catch your breath, then repeat. The time flies by, and the benefits add up!

Peak Intervals: What to Do

TIME	INTENSITY LEVEL
0:00–5:00	Warmup (see page 237).
5:01–6:00	Return to marching or jogging in place, swinging your arms at your sides. Walk or jog at an easy pace. If you're on a cardio machine, go at an easy pace. (If you're swimming, swim at an easy pace for 5 minutes.)
6:01–7:00	Level B (somewhat hard—you're breathing a bit harder, but you can talk in complete sentences).
7:01–25:00	Peak intervals. One interval is: • 15 seconds at Level D (breathless—you don't want to talk, but you could manage yes/no answers), followed by: • 45 seconds at Level B (somewhat hard). Repeat the full interval 18 times.
25:01–26:00	Level B.
26:01–30:00	Cooldown at Level A (easy—rhythmic breathing; you can sing).

Endurance Toning Routine

The second part of your Day 1 workout is your toning/strength-training routine. So pick up your weights and let's get started! For endurance toning, use lighter weights and do more reps.

Use a weight that you can lift at least 18 times. When you can easily do 22 reps, increase the amount of weight you're lifting. Aim to do 18 to 20 reps of each exercise, on each side when appropriate, at a moderate pace of about 1 count for each lifting and lowering phase of a move (unless otherwise noted).

Do the moves in the order listed. You can rest for 30 to 60 seconds (more if needed) between exercises. If you have time, repeat the series again.

TEST PANELIST TIP: *Adjust for Aches*

Recently diagnosed with osteoarthritis in her knee, Dale Honig also faced two other exercise challenges: sciatica and arthritis in the small of her back. A trainer at Rodale's fitness center suggested she adapt the 2-Day Diet strength-training moves to take pressure off her knees and back, so she does the exercises while sitting in a chair.

Nancy Barnes also modified the strength-training routine so it was easier on her knees. "Don't be discouraged if you can't do the moves a certain way," she says. "Adapt them and you'll still get a good workout."

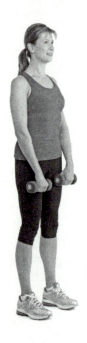
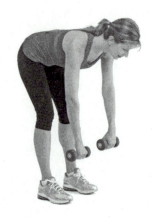
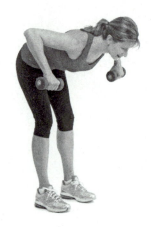

Hinge & Row

A. Stand with your feet about shoulder-width apart. Hold a dumbbell in each hand in front of your legs, palms facing thighs.

B. Keeping your abs tight, bend forward from your hips, sliding the weights down your thighs. Slowly lower (about 4 counts) until your torso is almost parallel to the floor. If you notice that your back is rounding

before that point, stop there. Dumbbells should be below your shoulders.

C. Bend your elbows toward the ceiling and pull the dumbbells up until your arms are bent at 90 degrees.

D. Straighten your arms. Do one more row, then slowly stand back up (4 counts). Repeat.

EASIER *(or if you have back problems): Hold on to the back of a chair with one hand and do one-arm rows.*

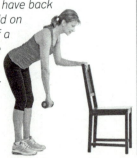

HARDER: *Do one-legged hinges. Let one leg lift behind you as you bend forward.*

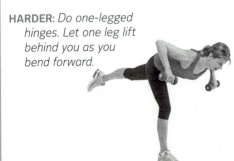

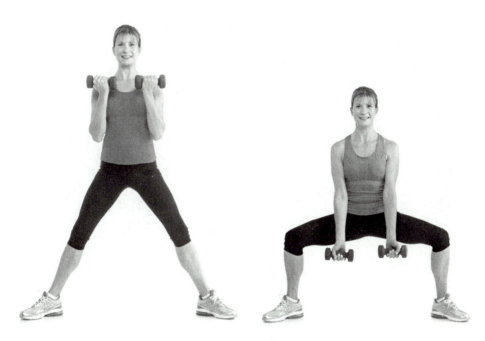

Plié Squat & Curl

A. Stand with your feet wider than shoulder-width apart, toes pointing out. Hold a dumbbell in each hand with arms bent so your hands are by your shoulders, palms facing you.

B. Keeping your abs tight, bend your knees and lower yourself until your thighs are almost parallel to the floor.

At the same time, straighten your arms and lower the dumbbells between your legs, palms facing forward.

C. Straighten your legs, squeeze your buttocks, and stand back up. Simultaneously, curl the dumbbells up toward your shoulders without moving your upper arms. Repeat.

EASIER: *Don't bend your knees as far.*

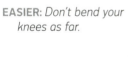
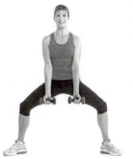

HARDER: *As you stand up, raise one foot off the floor to do a side knee lift.*

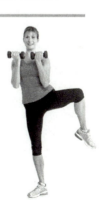

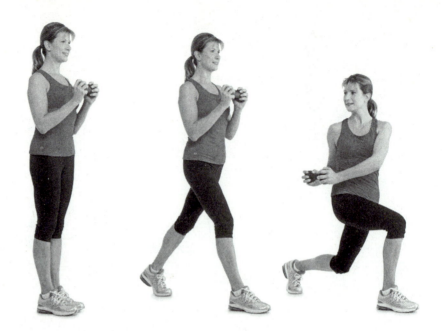

Lunge & Twist

A. Stand with your feet together. Hold a dumbbell with both hands and with arms bent so the dumbbell is in front of your chest.

B. Keeping your abs tight, step back with your left foot about 2 to 3 feet and bend your knees. Lower yourself until your right thigh is parallel to the floor, keeping your right knee above

your ankle. Your back heel will be off the floor. At the same time, rotate your torso to the right, bringing the dumbbell down by your right hip.

C. Press off your back foot to stand up as you rotate back to the start position. Repeat for the recommended number of reps, then switch sides.

EASIER: *Do stationary lunges, beginning with your feet apart and keeping them in that position the entire time.*

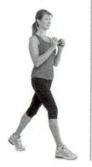

HARDER: *As you stand up, raise your back leg up in front of you to a knee lift.*

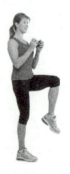

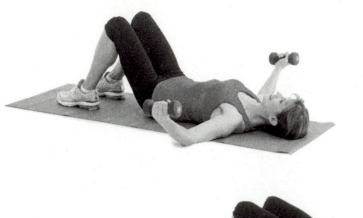

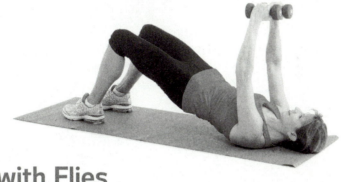

Bridge with Flies

A. Lie on your back with your legs bent and your feet flat on the floor. Hold a dumbbell in each hand with arms extended out to your sides, elbows slightly bent and palms facing up.

B. Squeeze your glutes and abs and lift your lower and middle back off the floor. At the same time, raise the dumbbells over your chest as if you were hugging a ball.

C. Lower your back and arms to the floor. Repeat.

EASIER: *Lift into the bridge first, then raise your arms. Lower your arms and back separately or at the same time, whichever is easier for you.*

HARDER: *Hold in the up position and raise one foot off the floor. Hold for a second, then lower your foot to the floor. Then lower your arms and back to the floor at the same time. Alternate legs with each rep.*

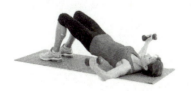

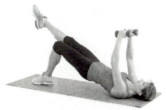

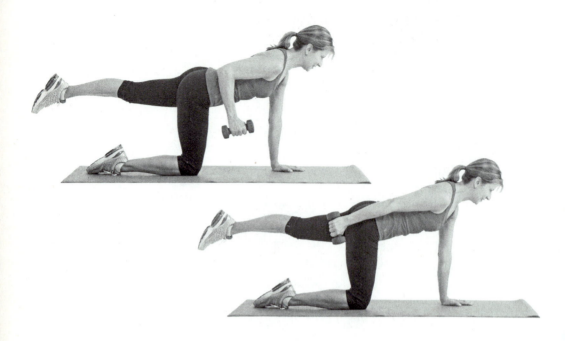

Kneeling Arm Raise

A. Get down on the floor on all fours. Hold a dumbbell in your right hand with your arm bent 90 degrees, your elbow by your hip, and your palm facing your thigh. Extend your left leg behind you and off the floor so you're balancing on your left hand and right knee. If your left wrist bothers you, hold a dumbbell so your wrist isn't bent.

B. Slowly straighten your right arm and raise the dumbbell behind you. Keep your abs tight and look at the floor a few feet in front of you to keep your head in line with your spine.

C. Slowly bend your arm back to the start position. Your upper arm should remain still throughout the move. Repeat for the recommended number of reps, then switch sides.

EASIER: *Keep both knees on the floor.*

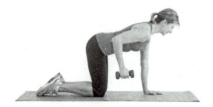

HARDER: *Bend and straighten your leg as you bend and straighten your arm.*

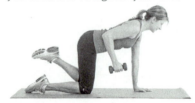

DAY 2: TEMPO INTERVAL WORKOUT PLUS POWER TONING ROUTINE

This routine boosts stamina, builds muscle, and burns calories so you're stronger, shapelier, and slimmer! You'll accomplish this with longer, lower-intensity intervals and with power toning using heavier weights during your strength-training session.

The Warmup

As with the Day 1 workout, your warmup is an important opportunity to prepare your muscles, joints, and connective tissue for the adventure ahead. Don't skimp—warming up will help you get more out of your routine, allow you to feel at your best as you exercise, and help lower your risk for injury.

Day 2: Warmup

TIME (MINUTES)	WHAT TO DO
0:00–1:00	March or jog in place, swinging your arms at your sides. Walk or jog at an easy pace. If you're on a cardio machine, go at an easy pace. (If you're swimming, swim at an easy pace for 5 minutes.)
1:01–2:00	While doing your activity from the first minute, reach both arms overhead 20 times. Pump your arms at your sides for the remaining time.
2:01–3:00	Keep moving your legs and press your arms in front of you at chest height, then pull them back so your elbows are pointing behind you, hands by your chest. Do 20 times. Pump your arms at your sides for the remaining time.
3:01–4:00	Keep moving your legs and alternately circle each arm backward, palm facing away from you. Do 40 circles total, 20 with each arm. Pump your arms at your sides for the remaining time.
4:01–5:00	Keep your legs moving and pump your arms at your sides.

Tempo Interval Workout

Tempo intervals are less intense than peak intervals. After your warmup, you'll alternate between Level B (somewhat hard) and Level C (hard).

You can do this routine with your favorite cardio workout.

Tempo Training

TIME (MINUTES)	WHAT TO DO
0:00–5:00	Warmup (see page 245).
5:01–6:00	Level B (somewhat hard—you are breathing a bit harder, but you can talk in complete sentences).
6:01–10:00	Level C (hard—you're slightly breathless and can talk only in brief phrases).
10:01–11:00	Level B.
11:01–15:00	Level C.
15:01–16:00	Level B.
16:01–20:00	Level C.
20:01–21:00	Level B.
21:01–25:00	Level C.
25:01–30:00	Cooldown at Level A (easy—rhythmic breathing; you can sing).

Power Toning Routine

For the Power Toning Routine, you'll do the same strength-building moves you learned for the Day 1 Endurance Toning Routine. The difference? Today you'll use heavier weights and do fewer reps.

Use a weight that you can lift only eight times. When you can easily do 12 reps, increase the amount of weight you're lifting. Aim to do 8 to 10 reps of each exercise, on each side when appropriate, at a slow pace of about 3 counts for each lifting and lowering phase of a move (unless otherwise noted).

Do the moves in the order listed. You can rest for 30 to 60 seconds (more if needed) between exercises. If you have time, repeat the series again.

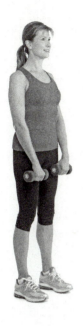
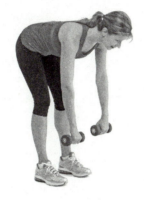
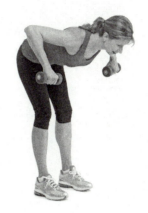

Hinge & Row

A. Stand with your feet about shoulder-width apart. Hold a dumbbell in each hand in front of your legs, palms facing thighs.

B. Keeping your abs tight, bend forward from your hips, sliding the weights down your thighs. Slowly lower yourself (about 4 counts) until your torso is almost parallel to the floor. If you notice that your back is rounding

before that point, stop there. Dumbbells should be below your shoulders.

C. Bend your elbows toward the ceiling and pull the dumbbells up until your arms are bent at 90 degrees.

D. Straighten your arms. Do one more row, then slowly stand back up (4 counts). Repeat.

EASIER *(or if you have back problems): Hold on to the back of a chair with one hand and do one-arm rows.*

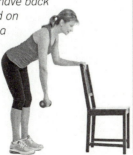

HARDER: *Do one-legged hinges. Let one leg lift behind you as you bend forward.*

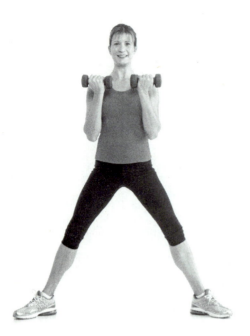
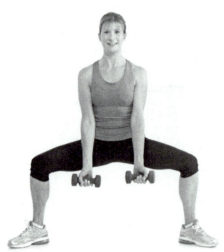

Plié Squat & Curl

A. Stand with your feet wider than shoulder-width apart, toes pointing out. Hold a dumbbell in each hand with arms bent so your hands are by your shoulders, palms facing you.

B. Keeping your abs tight, bend your knees and lower yourself until your thighs are almost parallel to the floor. At the same time, straighten your arms and lower the dumbbells between your legs, palms facing forward.

C. Straighten your legs, squeeze your buttocks, and stand back up. Simultaneously, curl the dumbbells up toward your shoulders without moving your upper arms. Repeat.

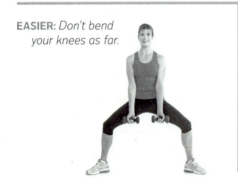

EASIER: *Don't bend your knees as far.*

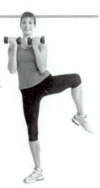

HARDER: *As you stand up, raise one foot off the floor to do a side knee lift.*

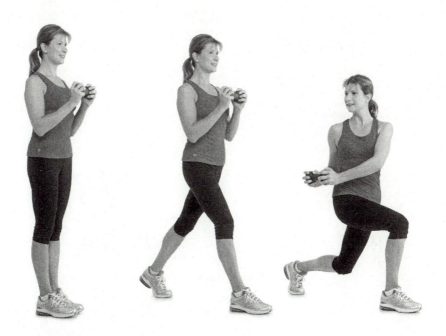

Lunge & Twist

A. Stand with your feet together. Hold a dumbbell with both hands and with arms bent so the dumbbell is in front of your chest.

B. Keeping your abs tight, step back with your left foot about 2 to 3 feet and bend your knees. Lower yourself until your right thigh is parallel to the floor, keeping your right knee above

your ankle. Your back heel will be off the floor. At the same time, rotate your torso to the right, bringing the dumbbell down by your right hip.

C. Press off your back foot to stand up as you rotate back to the start position. Repeat for the recommended number of reps, then switch sides.

EASIER: *Do stationary lunges, beginning with your feet apart and keeping them in that position the entire time.*

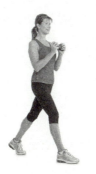

HARDER: *As you stand up, raise your back leg up in front of you to a knee lift.*

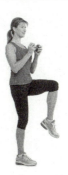

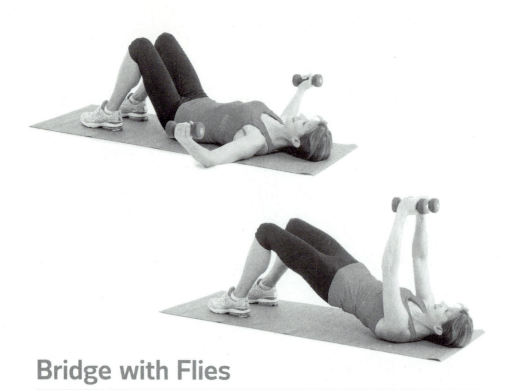

Bridge with Flies

A. Lie on your back with your legs bent and your feet flat on the floor. Hold a dumbbell in each hand with your arms extended out to your sides, elbows slightly bent and palms facing up.

B. Squeeze your glutes and abs and lift your lower and middle back off the floor. At the same time, raise the dumbbells over your chest as if you were hugging a ball.

C. Lower your back and arms to the floor. Repeat.

EASIER: Lift into the bridge first, then raise your arms. Lower your arms and back separately or at the same time, whichever is easier for you.

HARDER: Hold in the up position and raise one foot off the floor. Hold for a second, then lower your foot to the floor. Then lower your arms and back to the floor at the same time. Alternate legs each rep.

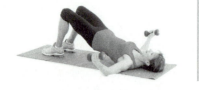

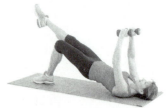

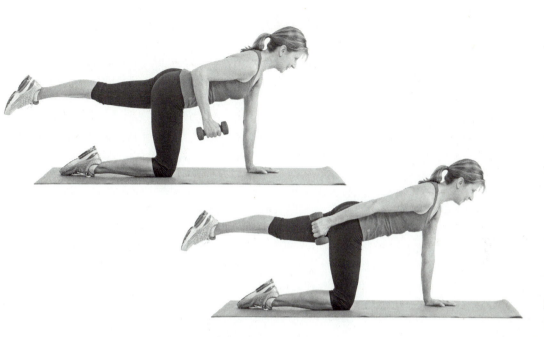

Kneeling Arm Raise

A. Get down on the floor on all fours. Hold a dumbbell in your right hand with your arm bent 90 degrees, your elbow by your hip, and your palm facing your thigh. Extend your left leg behind you and off the floor so you're balancing on your left hand and right knee. If your left wrist bothers you, hold a dumbbell so your wrist isn't bent.

B. Slowly straighten your right arm and raise the dumbbell behind you. Keep your abs tight and look at the floor a few feet in front of you to keep your head in line with your spine.

C. Slowly bend your arm back to the start position. Your upper arm should remain still throughout the move. Repeat for the recommended number of reps, then switch sides.

EASIER: *Keep both knees on the floor.*

HARDER: *Bend and straighten your leg as you bend and straighten your arm.*

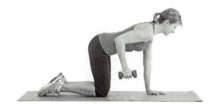

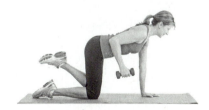

Sharon Spitz

AGE: 38

HEIGHT: 5'3½"

POUNDS LOST: Lost 7.8 pounds of body fat and gained 8.8 pounds of muscle

INCHES LOST: 7, including 0.5 inch from her waist and 2 inches from each thigh

HEALTH UPGRADE: Her LDL cholesterol fell 29 points.

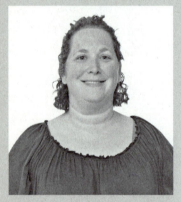

BEFORE

Motivated to Move!

As a registered nurse who works in corporate health for a large manufacturing company, Sharon Spitz knew that eating breakfast was a basic tenet of good health. But as the mom of 4-year-old twins, breakfast was just something else to fit in to her hectic mornings. And often she didn't—until the 2-Day Diet.

"I've added breakfast to my lifestyle now," she says. "I don't want to feel so hungry that I'm starving at lunch, and I like having more energy throughout the morning. Since I was eating low-carb and needed to eat in the car on the way to work, I went with low-fat cheese or celery and peanut butter. They taste good, but unlike cereal, there are no crumbs in my car!"

Mission accomplished. Despite a busy work schedule that keeps her traveling several days a week—and in spite of a 2-week overseas vacation for a family wedding in the middle of the diet—Sharon was impressed by her results. "Weight is just a number—it doesn't tell you anything about what's happening inside your body," she says. "I'm happy that my body fat went down and my lean muscle increased. As you gain muscle, you get healthier, so that's important. My LDL cholesterol went down, too, which made me happy. There's heart disease in my family, and I'd like to avoid that."

The fact that Sharon gained a pound but lost inches is a testament to the fact that muscle takes less room than fat. "Losing inches is part of the real success picture," she says. "My clothes fit better, and I feel good. That's what counts."

The entire time she was on the diet, she never felt she was giving up the foods she likes. "All of us really enjoyed the Beef and Scallion Stir-Fry," she says. "And my husband and I liked the Chef Salad Wrap,

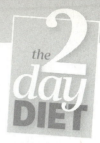

too." Family food allergies and preferences meant she kept nuts out of family meals and often used chicken in place of pork in recipes. "The meals were easy and healthy," she says. "Years ago we had tried another low-carb diet plan, and the foods were very high in fat. On that plan, my husband made a soup so thick the spoon stood up—it was full of butter! I was working in a hospital cardiac unit at the time and knew that wasn't a good idea. The 2-Day Diet is different. And the flexibility means it's easy to recover from an 'oops' day."

But how did Sharon gain all that muscle? A combination of low-carb eating, shown to help maintain muscle mass and help muscle cells burn more fuel, and the 2-Day Diet Workout. Sharon faithfully trekked to the company gym several days a week, where she performed the workout's toning routine and did intervals on her favorite piece of gym equipment, the elliptical trainer. She'd punch up music or a National Public Radio podcast on her mp3 player to make the time fly.

"This program really enhanced my exercise routine," she says. "It encouraged me to work out more often and to work out smarter. I feel stronger and have more endurance now."

Sharon joined lunchtime soccer games with her co-workers, too. "Before, I would've been worn out after 10 minutes. Now I can play longer and have fun," she says. She's glad her kids have an active mom as a role model. "If your children see you sitting a lot, they'll want to sit, too." she says. "I want them to be active for life—so that physical activity is second nature to them. It's part of my motivation to keep on exercising."

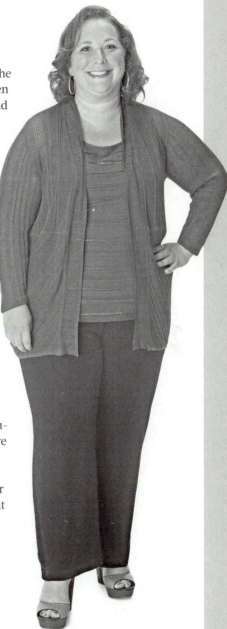

PART IV

Tools and

Congratulations! You've done it. You've followed the 2-Day Diet, you've trimmed pounds and inches, and now you're enjoying a slimmer, healthier, more energetic you.

Every single one of our test panelists reported that they felt better after just 6 weeks on the 2-Day Diet—and all you have to do is look at their before-and-after photos, scattered throughout this book, to see that they looked better, too. Dropping a size or two, fitting into old clothes or buying new outfits, enjoying a bounce in energy and a spring in their steps . . . all our participants agreed: The 2-Day Diet was a great success. Just ask Kathy Rocchetti. She fit back into her "skinny" jeans and reveled in compliments from family and friends. "People who hadn't seen me in a while would come up to me and say, 'Wow, you look great! Something's really changed about you.' Actually, lots of things have changed. My aches and pains have disappeared, my skin's cleared up, and I have a much more positive attitude. This diet has become a way of life for me. Not only has it made me healthier, it's boosted my confidence."

Resources

But even though Kathy's 2-Day Diet was a great success, she knows that it was just part of her journey. Turning the plan from a diet into a way of life is the next step. In this section, we'll show you how to maintain—and build on—your weight-loss accomplishments and your health improvements. You'll find dozens of practical guidelines and lots of great advice for keeping those pounds off for good.

From eating mindfully to rewarding yourself for your victories and forgiving yourself those inevitable little slipups, you'll find a handy tool kit to help you stay slim and trim forever. And be sure to check out even more resources at the back of the book. In Appendix A, beginning on page 275, you'll find a handy chart with nutritional values for just about any food you can think of to help you build your own delicious, healthy meals. And in Appendix B, starting on page 291, you'll find 3 weeks' worth of journal pages that you're free to photocopy, to help you track your eating and your exercise.

So give yourself one more pat on the back—then try our strategies for continued success. We wish you all the best as you embark on your continuing journey!

after the diet: Keeping the Weight Off

Hooray! You've done it! After 6 weeks on the 2-Day Diet, you've lost pounds and inches. Your clothes are feeling a bit loose—perhaps you've had to take in the waistband on your pants and skirts, haul out smaller clothes that had gone into storage, or even shop for a new wardrobe. You've got new energy and newfound confidence. Your skin glows, and people around you see the change in you. Congratulations!

Now it's time to maintain your new weight and your new shape. And the good news is that the 2-Day Diet gives you the tools you need to do just that—and to sidestep the weight regain that disappoints so many people on conventional diet plans. The 2-Day Diet won't just drop you off at the end of your weight-loss journey, leaving you to fend for yourself in a world full of tempting high-calorie food, big portions, and busy days that don't easily allow time for exercise. Here's how you can use the 2-Day Diet to keep weight off, nip regain in the bud, and defend your trimmer, healthier body during the most calorie-intensive times of the year—like holidays, vacations, and special occasions. It worked for our test panelists and will work for you, too!

STRATEGY #1: MAKE REGULAR-CARB MEALS YOUR EVERYDAY DIET

The 5 days a week of healthy regular-carb meals that you enjoyed on the 2-Day Diet deliver balanced nutrition and a satisfying mix of lean protein, good fats, fruits, veggies, whole grains, and dairy. These are the foods that belong on your plate every day. You're already a pro at this way of eating, so why not make this your go-to eating plan from now on?

Plan on having 2 to 3 servings of fruit; 4 to 6 servings of vegetables; 3 to 7 servings of whole grains, starchy vegetables, and/or dried beans; 2 to 3 servings of low-fat or fat-free dairy products; 2 to 3 servings of healthy fats (such as olive or canola oil, nuts, and avocado); and 2 to 3 servings of lean protein a day. Or make it easy and use the "plate method" for perfect portion control and a healthy balance of foods: Reserve half of your plate for produce, one-fourth for grains, and one-fourth for lean protein—then just add dairy and good fats as described.

STRATEGY #2: STICK WITH THE 2-DAY DIET WORKOUT

No other exercise program fits this easily into your day or delivers these kinds of results! The interval-training routines take just a half hour twice a week and burn more calories and more body fat than steady-paced exercise, so make this your go-to workout every week! Add the 2-Diet Workout's toning/strength-training

TEST PANELIST TIP: *Find Pockets of Downtime*

With three busy children ages 8, 10, and 12, a household to manage, and a part-time job as an exercise instructor, Karen Fazioli takes advantage of little pockets of spare time to fit in her own exercise routine.

"I walk around the sidelines at my daughter's field hockey practices or take a walk when my son's at a fencing lesson," she says. "I do my weight routine while watching TV at night."

Splitting up your workout makes fitting it in a snap. You can do the intervals at one time and the strength moves at another, or even split up the strength-training routine into tiny stretches of free time. Paula Weiant did part of the 2-Day Diet strength-training program a couple of minutes before going to work in the morning, and the rest after she got home at night.

moves, which take just 15 minutes twice a week. These multitasking, multi-muscle moves help maintain and build muscle, which will help your body burn more calories round the clock—a "secret weapon" for maintaining your new weight!

STRATEGY #3: EAT LOW-CARB AS NEEDED TO KEEP WEIGHT OFF

Should you keep on eating low-carb? That's up to you. Test panelists fit in extra low-carb days to balance out times when they expected to eat more—like on vacation, at weddings, and over holiday weekends. It worked! In one British study of part-time low-carb dieting, volunteers kept eating low-carb 1 day a week for a month after they'd lost weight. The researchers expected that this strategy would help them maintain their weight loss, but the study volunteers actually continued to lose weight![1]

You can also bring back low-carb eating 1 or 2 days a week if you notice you've gained a little weight or if you'd like a little extra weight-loss oomph before bathing suit season or in the months and weeks leading up to a big event when you want to look your best. It couldn't be simpler!

FOUR MIND TRICKS FOR EVEN EASIER MAINTENANCE

There's a certain excitement that can inspire you to stick with a successful weight-loss diet: The number on the scale keeps dropping, you fit into favorite clothes that had become too tight to wear, your family and friends tell you how great you look. But we'll be honest. In contrast, maintaining a new, lower weight often doesn't feel as thrilling. It should. But it's easy to take your new weight or

TEST PANELIST TIP: *Fitting in Office Treats*

From birthday cake and doughnuts to pizza lunches, office food is the downfall of many diets. But Mary Banyas discovered that approaching these temptations in a new way allowed her to stay on track. "I missed bagels," she says. "Sometimes I'd smell one toasting at work, so on a regular-carb day, I might have just a quarter of a bagel. And every month, we have a party to celebrate all the birthdays of the month. Last month, I had just one slice of pizza plus a big salad and a tiny piece of cake."

slimmer hips for granted. What helps keep the excitement high—and keep your head in the weight-maintaining game?

Researchers from Penn State Hershey Medical Center had the same question. They surveyed 1,200 successful dieters and discovered that those who'd kept off their weight for at least 12 months had hit on some mind tricks that spelled success. They kept on choosing lean proteins, for example, along with their fruit, vegetables, and whole grains. They kept on exercising. And they adopted wise mental/emotional strategies. They rewarded themselves for staying on track—but not with food. And they gave themselves regular pep talks.[2]

British researchers found even more clues about the habits of successful weight maintainers when they studied 28 women who'd regained lost weight, 28 who'd maintained a new lower weight, and 20 who'd stayed at a stable weight. Among the great mental traits of maintainers: They were thrilled at their new weight, instead of feeling discouraged that they hadn't lost even more. They forgave themselves and moved on when they slipped up, instead of letting one brownie or ice-cream cone lead them down the road back to overeating.[3]

Still more clues come from the National Weight Control Registry, a data bank of valuable information about people who've lost a significant amount of weight and kept it off. Researchers discovered that successful maintainers had lower stress levels than people who relapsed and regained. Regainers' tension levels were about 20 percent higher, and stress made them more likely to stop trying to maintain their weight once they slipped up.[4]

What does all of that research mean for you? Simply that these mind tricks can help you stay slimmer:

1. **Reward yourself generously.** Your new jeans still fit? The bathroom scale reports you're at the same weight as last week? This calls for a celebration! No, not a piece of cake. Reward yourself richly—with a special walk, a movie, a new music download for your mp3 player, even that new top or dress you noticed in the catalog that just arrived. Rewards don't have to be large or expensive. What counts is that they make you feel good and that you reward yourself regularly for staying on track.

2. **Dare to love your new size.** In that British study, women who put weight back on had never felt satisfied with their weight loss or their new shape. One even told researchers that she felt okay at first, then "started feeling fat again." In contrast, one maintainer felt absolutely "jubilant." Achieving this positive state of mind lets you reverse negative self-criticism about

your body. That's a great thing! It also means not allowing yourself to blame your size or weight for other issues in your life—like boredom or disappointment. Spend some time appreciating your new shape. Dress it well. Take care of it. Repeat often.

3. **Don't let a slip become a slide.** What if you do regain a pound or two or discover that you somehow ordered a large ice-cream sundae with three toppings and ate the whole thing? Take a deep breath, acknowledge that everyone slips up, then get back to healthy eating—or get back to a day or two of low-carb eating to reverse the regain. Adopting a flexible, accepting attitude will do more to help you stay slim than all-or-nothing thinking can, the British researchers say.

4. **Make time to unwind.** Stress eating is wired into our brains. Tension makes us crave high-fat, high-carb foods and stores the extra calories at your midsection. Your best antidote? De-stress regularly in whatever way makes you feel great. Call a friend, walk the dog, do some deep-breathing exercises, do a little yoga, write in your journal, meditate . . . it's all good— and good for you.

TEST PANELIST TIP: *Join a Class*

Plenty of classes deliver the high- and low-intensity mix plus toning, strength-building moves that you'll also find in the 2-Day Diet Workout.

"I walked a lot when I started the 2-Day Diet, then I incorporated the weight routine and really saw results," says Anne Marie York. "To stay motivated, I joined a class at my gym. We did the same kinds of strength-training exercises as in the 2-Day Diet Workout."

Dale Honig takes a "hydrobike" class at her local gym: Participants do a spinning routine on specially designed bikes that sit in a pool—a great workout that's easy on knees and hips, while burning calories and building cardiovascular fitness with interval work. Her class kept her accountable, she says: "I do better in a class than disciplining myself to do it at home."

Mary Banyas signed up for a Zumba class close to home. "I have so much more energy now," she says. "I feel really great!"

MAINTAIN YOUR HEALTH

Dropping those pounds has been great for your looks—but even better for your health. All our test panelists reported improvements in a variety of measures, from lower blood pressure to lower cholesterol and lower triglycerides. But a recent study showed that maintaining that weight loss is super-important for continued good health. One hundred twelve women took part in a 5-month weight-loss plan, shedding an average of 25 pounds each. But after 1 year, two-thirds of the women regained about 70 percent of their lost weight. And researchers found that for those regainers, several of their risk factors for cardiovascular health were worse than they were before their weight loss. (On the other hand, those who maintained their weight continued to enjoy improvements in heart health.)[5]

All the more reason to focus on maintaining your weight loss.

IT WORKS!

You *can* keep the weight off. Just follow the example of test panelist Dale Honig. She lost 12.8 pounds in 6 weeks on the 2-Day Diet, but she didn't stop there. Dale kept on following the program and lost an additional 7.2 pounds! "I went to have my 6-month checkup this week," she told us in late August 2012, "and my doctor was amazed that I am 20 pounds lighter since my last visit in March. My blood pressure was the lowest since my annual checkup, at 118/68." She plans to keep going and trim a few more pounds. "It's making a big difference in my life!" she says.

SUCCESS STORY:
Anne Marie York

AGE: 51

HEIGHT: 5'6"

POUNDS LOST: 6.8, including 4.6 pounds of body fat

INCHES LOST: 17.75, including 4 inches from her waist and 3.75 inches from her hips

HEALTH UPGRADE: Her blood pressure and triglycerides fell to healthier levels; her LDL cholesterol dropped 25 points.

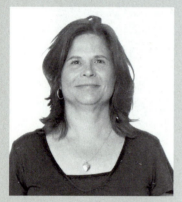

BEFORE

Healthy for Life!

Losing inches opened up a whole new world of clothes for Anne Marie York—and they were waiting for her right upstairs in her own attic. "A few weeks into the 2-Day Diet, I was looking through an old bin in my attic that was full of clothes I used to wear," she says. "I found a pair of beautiful dressy capri pants I'd bought 6 years ago to wear to my niece's graduation. They haven't fit me since, but now they did again! I wore them to work on a hot day and got lots of compliments."

For Anne Marie, the 2-Day Diet reinforced healthy eating and exercise habits she had already put in place. "I keep grilled chicken and steak in my refrigerator for quick meals," she says. "On the diet, though, I made sure I had them with salad or a vegetable. I think this is a healthy way of eating for life, not just something you do for 6 weeks and then stop."

A medical supplies manager for a hospital, Anne Marie stuck with healthy eating and regular exercise even during a hectic period when the hospital opened two new departments. Her secret weapon? Packing her own lunch and snacks and toting them along with her. "There's food everywhere at work, and it's not always the healthiest," she says. "But as long as I have food with me that I know I can eat, I won't go into one of the snack bars or the cafeteria or the gift shop to pick something up. I'll think twice about spending the money and eating all those extra carbs."

In her lunch bag now: cottage cheese and fruit; cheese and turkey pepperoni ("I used to eat those with crackers. Now I eat them plain," she says.); hummus and carrots; celery or rice cakes with

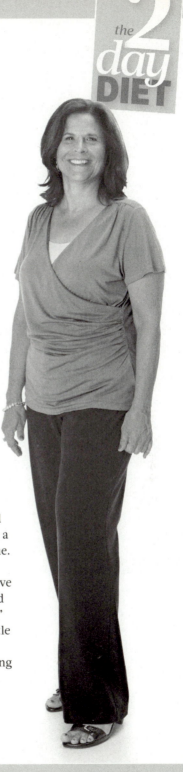

almond butter. "I'll have eggs and bacon or a meal replacement bar for breakfast," she says. "Today I had a burger—no bun—with veggies and hummus for lunch. I was good till late afternoon, when I had some cottage cheese. This is a plan I can stick with for a long time!"

She loved choosing her own low-carb days and the wide variety of foods on the plan. "I quickly saw that having my choice of days to go low-carb was big. Weekdays were better for me for that. I'm more in a routine," she says. Making adjustments was easy, too. "If I have too many carbs at a meal, I'll kick it back up at the next meal or start again the next day. I loved that about this plan. I don't want to have somebody tell me what I can and cannot eat. When you get to a certain age and have done this so many times, you don't want to be restricted anymore."

Getting out of what she calls the "carb rut" made longtime chocolate cravings vanish. "I used to eat chocolate every day," she says. "I still like it a lot, but I don't feel like I have to have it all the time. I was just on a vacation and had some chocolate-covered almonds. They were good, but I didn't have to have any more chocolate." And she's discovered a new favorite: mashed cauliflower. "It's so good," she says. "You just steam it and mash it with a little milk and butter. It's amazing." The best thing about the 2-Day Diet? For Anne Marie, it's knowing that she's got a plan she can turn to for life—no matter what life throws her way. "I love knowing I can restart the low-carb days to help me if I gain a few pounds or want to lose more weight."

ENDNOTES

Chapter 1. The 2-Day Diet: Easiest Weight Loss Ever!

1. M. N. Harvie et al. "Intermittent Dietary Carbohydrate Restriction Enables Weight Loss and Reduces Breast Cancer Risk Biomarkers." Presented at the CTRC-AACR San Antonio Breast Cancer Symposium, December 2011.
2. E. L. Weinheimer et al. "A Systematic Review of the Separate and Combined Effects of Energy Restriction and Exercise on Fat-Free Mass in Middle-Aged and Older Adults: Implications for Sarcopenic Obesity." *Nutrition Reviews* 68, no. 7 (July 2010): 375–88.
3. A. H. Manninen. "Metabolic Advantage of Low-Carbohydrate Diets: A Calorie Is Still Not a Calorie." *American Journal of Clinical Nutrition* 83, no. 6 (June 2006): 1442–43.
4. C. B. Ebbling. "Effects of Dietary Composition on Energy Expenditure during Weight-Loss Maintenance." *Journal of the American Medical Association* 307, no. 24 (June 2012): 2627–34.

Chapter 2. Weight-Loss Power

1. Garfield G. Duncan. "Intermittent Fasts in the Correction and Control of Intractable Obesity." *Transactions of the American Clinical and Climatological Association* 74 (1963): 121–29.
2. K. A. Varady. "Do Calorie Restriction or Alternate-Day Fasting Regimens Modulate Adipose Tissue Physiology in a Way That Reduces Chronic Disease Risk?" *Nutrition Reviews* 66, no. 6 (2008): 333–42.
3. R. M. Anson. "Intermittent Fasting Dissociates Beneficial Effects of Dietary Restriction on Glucose Metabolism and Neuronal Resistance to Injury from Calorie Intake." *Proceedings of the National Academy of Sciences* 100, no. 10 (2003): 6216–20.

4. K. Vondra. "Effect of Protracted Intermittent Fasting on the Activities of Enzymes Involved in Energy Metabolism, and on the Concentrations of Glycogen, Protein and DNA in Skeletal Muscle of Obese Women." *Nutrition and Metabolism* 20, no. 5 (1976): 329–37.

5. E. A. Vallejo. "Hunger Diet on Alternate Days in the Nutrition of the Aged." *PrensaMedica Argentina* 44, no. 2 (1957): 119–20.

6. R. M. Karns. "Dramatic Treatment for Obesity: Diseased Patients Test Starvation Diet." *Journal of the American Medical Association* 197, no. S1 (1966): S1–22.

7. L. K. Heilbronn. "Glucose Tolerance and Skeletal Muscle Gene Expression in Response to Alternate Day Fasting." *Obesity Research* 13, no. 3 (2005): 574–81.

8. ———. "Alternate-Day Fasting in Nonobese Subjects: Effects on Body Weight, Body Composition, and Energy Metabolism." *American Journal of Clinical Nutrition* 81 (2005): 69–73.

9. N. Halberg et al. "Effect of Intermittent Fasting and Refeeding on Insulin Action in Healthy Men." *Journal of Applied Physiology* 99 (2005): 2128–36.

10. J. B. Johnson et al. "Alternate Day Calorie Restriction Improves Clinical Findings and Reduces Markers of Oxidative Stress and Inflammation in Overweight Adults with Moderate Asthma." *Free Radical Biology & Medicine* 42 (2007): 665–74.

11. K. A. Varady et al. "Short-Term Modified Alternate-Day Fasting: A Novel Dietary Strategy for Weight Loss and Cardioprotection in Obese Adults." *American Journal of Clinical Nutrition* 90 (2009): 1138–43.

12. M. N. Harvie et al. "The Effects of Intermittent or Continuous Energy Restriction on Weight Loss and Metabolic Disease Risk Markers: A Randomized Trial in Young Overweight Women." *International Journal of Obesity* 35, no. 5 (2011): 714–27.

13. Harvie et al. "Intermittent Dietary Carbohydrate Restriction."

14. Johns Hopkins University. "Losing Belly Fat, Whether from a Low-Carb or a Low-Fat Diet, Helps Improve Blood Vessel Function." Accessed March 13, 2012, www.hopkinsmedicine.org/news/media/releases/losing_belly_fat_whether_from_a_low_carb_or_a_low_fat_diet_helps_improve_blood_vessel_function.

15. Ebbling. "Effects of Dietary Composition on Energy Expenditure."

16. J. D. Browning et al. "Alterations in Hepatic Glucose and Energy Metabolism as a Result of Calorie and Carbohydrate Restriction." *Hepatology* 48, no. 5 (2008): 1487–96.

17. L. L. Goree et al. "Effects of Dietary Macronutrient Composition on Total and Intra-Abdominal Adipose Tissue during Weight Maintenance and

Weight Loss." *Endocrine Reviews* 32 (03_MeetingAbstracts) (June 2011): 2-459.

18. R. R. Wing and R. W. Jeffrey. "Prescribed 'Breaks' as a Means to Disrupt Weight Control Efforts." *Obesity Research* 11 (2003): 287–91.

19. A. M. Johnstone. "Effects of a High-Protein Ketogenic Diet on Hunger, Appetite, and Weight Loss in Obese Men Feeding Ad Libitum." *American Journal of Clinical Nutrition* 87, no. 1 (2008): 44–55.

20. The Endocrine Society. "Moderately Reduced Carbohydrate Diet Keeps People Feeling Full Longer." Accessed June 12, 2009, http://www.endo-society.org/media/ENDO-09/Moderatelyreducedcarbohydrate.cfm.

21. P. J. Enriori et al. "Leptin Resistance and Obesity," supplement, *Obesity* 14, no. S8 (August 2006): S254–S58.

22. K. A. Varady. "Intermittent versus Daily Calorie Restriction: Which Diet Regimen Is More Effective for Weight Loss?" *Obesity Reviews* 12, no. 7 (2011): 593–601.

23. Wayne Westcott. "ACSM Strength Training Guidelines: Role in Body Composition and Health Enhancement." *ACSM's Health & Fitness Journal* 13, no. 4 (2009).

24. Ibid.

Chapter 3. Health Power

1. Scott Grundy et al. "Implications of Recent Clinical Trials for the National Cholesterol Education Program Adult Treatment Panel III Guidelines." *Circulation* 110, no. 2 (2004): 227–39.

2. Mayo Clinic. "Mayo Clinic Releases Book with Action Plan to Help Beat Heart Disease." Press release, January 30, 2012. http://www.mayoclinic.org/news2012-rst/6680.html.

3. Graham A. Colditz. "Applying What We Know to Accelerate Cancer Prevention." *Science Translational Medicine* 4, no. 127 (2012): 127rv4.

4. F. B. Hu et al. "Diet, Lifestyle, and the Risk of Type 2 Diabetes Mellitus in Women." *New England Journal of Medicine* 345 (2001): 790–97.

5. www.nature.com/oby/journal/v16/n12/full/oby2008418a.html.

6. W. Yancy. "A Randomized Trial of a Low-Carbohydrate Diet vs. Orlistat plus a Low-Fat Diet for Weight Loss." *Archives of Internal Medicine* 170 (January 2010): 136–45.

7. Iris Shai et al. "Weight Loss with a Low-Carbohydrate, Mediterranean, or Low-Fat Diet." *New England Journal of Medicine* 359 (July 2008): 229–41.

8. T. Fung et al. "Low-Carbohydrate Diets and All-Cause and Cause-Specific

Mortality: Two Cohort Studies." *Annals of Internal Medicine* 153, no. 5 (2010): 289–98.

9. Ingegerd Johansson et al. "Associations among 25-Year Trends in Diet, Cholesterol and BMI from 140,000 Observations in Men and Women in Northern Sweden." *Nutrition Journal* 11, no. 1 (2012): 40.

10. D. J. A. Jenkins et al. "Effect of a Dietary Portfolio of Cholesterol-Lowering Foods Given at 2 Levels of Intensity of Dietary Advice on Serum Lipids in Hyperlipidemia: A Randomized Controlled Trial." *Journal of the American Medical Association* 306, no. 8 (2011): 831–39.

11. Harvie et al. "Intermittent Dietary Carbohydrate Restriction."

12. Ebbling. "Effects of Dietary Composition on Energy Expenditure."

13. Ahmad Esmaillzadeh et al. "Fruit and Vegetable Intakes, C-Reactive Protein, and the Metabolic Syndrome." *American Journal of Clinical Nutrition* 84, no. 6 (December 2006): 1489–97.

14. F. Hu. "Plant-Based Foods and Prevention of Cardiovascular Disease: An Overview," supplement, *American Journal of Clinical Nutrition* 78, no. S3 (2003): S544–S51.

15. Ibid.

16. Harvie et al. "The Effects of Intermittent or Continuous Energy Restriction."

17. M. J. Bonorden et al. "Intermittent Calorie Restriction Delays Prostate Tumor Detection and Increases Survival Time in TRAMP Mice." *Nutrition and Cancer* 61, no. 2 (2009): 265–75.

18. Varady et al. "Short-Term Modified Alternate-Day Fasting."

19. Cholesterol Treatment Trialists' (CTT) Collaborators. "Efficacy and Safety of Cholesterol-Lowering Treatment: Prospective Meta-Analysis of Data from 90,056 Participants in 14 Randomised Trials of Statins." *Lancet* 366, no. 9493 (2005): 1267–78.

20. Harvie et al. "The Effects of Intermittent or Continuous Energy Restriction."

21. Erin White. "On Track to Getting Even Fatter: By 2020 Majority of Adults in America Will Be Overweight, Suffer from Diabetic Conditions." Northwestern University News Center: November 16, 2011. www.northwestern.edu/newscenter/stories/2011/11/heart-health-fatter.html.

22. D. R. Jacobs et al. "Whole-Grain Consumption Is Associated with a Reduced Risk of Noncardiovascular, Noncancer Death Attributed to Inflammatory Diseases in the Iowa Women's Health Study." *American Journal of Clinical Nutrition* 85 (2007): 1606–14.

23. P. B. Mellen. "Whole Grain Intake and Cardiovascular Disease: A Meta-Analysis." *Nutrition, Metabolism & Cardiovascular Diseases* 18, no. 4 (2008): 283–90.

24. J. S. L. de Munter. "Whole Grain, Bran, and Germ Intake and Risk of Type 2 Diabetes: A Prospective Cohort Study and Systematic Review." *PLOS Medicine* 4, no. 8 (2007): e261.

25. Earl S. Ford et al. "Metabolic Syndrome and Risk of Incident Diabetes: Findings from the European Prospective Investigation into Cancer and Nutrition-Potsdam Study." *Cardiovascular Diabetology* 7 (2008): 35.

26. A. Galassi "Metabolic Syndrome and Risk of Cardiovascular Disease: A Meta-analysis." *American Journal of Medicine* 119, no. 10 (2006): 812–19.

27. D. Sharma et al. "Leptin Promotes the Proliferative Response and Invasiveness in Human Endometrial Cancer Cells by Activating Multiple Signal-Transduction Pathways." *Endocrine-Related Cancer* 13, no. 2 (2006): 629–40.

28. S. Guo et al. "Oncogenic Role and Therapeutic Target of Leptin Signaling in Breast Cancer and Cancer Stem Cells." *Biochimica et Biophysica Acta* 1825, no. 2 (2012): 207–22.

29. I. Barone et al. "Leptin Mediates Tumor-Stromal Interactions That Promote the Invasive Growth of Breast Cancer Cells." *Cancer Research* 72 (March 2012): 1416.

30. S. Catalano. "The Multifactorial Role of Leptin in Driving the Breast Cancer Microenvironment." *Nature Reviews Endocrinology* 8 (May 2012): 263–75.

31. B. Draznin. "Mechanism of the Mitogenic Influence of Hyperinsulinemia." *Diabetology & Metabolic Syndrome* 3 (2011): 10.

32. C. L. Thompson et al. "Insulin Resistance, Central Obesity, and Risk of Colorectal Adenomas." *Cancer* 118, no. 7 (2012): 1774–81.

33. M. J. Gunter. "Insulin, Insulin-Like Growth Factor-I, and Risk of Breast Cancer in Postmenopausal Women." *Journal of the National Cancer Institute* 101, no. 1 (2009): 48–60.

34. P. J. Goodwin et al. "Insulin- and Obesity-Related Variables in Early-Stage Breast Cancer: Correlations and Time Course of Prognostic Associations." *Journal of Clinical Oncology* 30, no. 2 (2012): 164–71.

35. Monica Bartucci et al. "Obesity Hormone Leptin Induces Growth and Interferes with the Cytotoxic Effects of 5-Fluorouracil in Colorectal Tumor Stem Cells." *Endocrine-Related Cancer* 17 (September 2010): 823–33.

36. R. W. Engelman et al. "Calorie Consumption Level Influences Development of C3H/Ou Breast Adenocarcinoma with Indifference to Calorie Source." *Proceedings of the Society for Experimental Biology and Medicine* 193, no. 1 (1990): 23–30.

37. American Association for Cancer Research. "Intermittent, Low-Carbohydrate

Diets More Successful Than Standard Dieting, Present Possible Intervention for Breast Cancer Prevention." Press release, December 11, 2011. http://www.aacr.org/home/public—media/aacr-press-releases.aspx?d=2649.

38. C. A. Befort et al. "Outcomes of a Weight Loss Intervention among Rural Breast Cancer Survivors." *Breast Cancer Research and Treatment* 132, no. 2 (2012): 631–39.

Chapter 4. Exercise Power

1. Centers for Disease Control and Prevention. "How Much Physical Activity Do Adults Need?" http://www.cdc.gov/physicalactivity/everyone/guidelines/adults.html.

2. The Gallup-Healthways Well-Being Index. May 29, 2012. www.gallup.com/poll/118570/nearly-half-exercise-less-three-days-week.aspx?version=print.

3. Caroline Richardson et al. "A Meta-Analysis of Pedometer-Based Walking Interventions and Weight Loss." *Annals of Family Medicine* 6 (2008): 69–77.

4. R. T. Clinghan. "Do You Get Value for Money When You Buy an Expensive Pair of Running Shoes?" *British Journal of Sports Medicine* 42, no. 3 (2007): 189–93.

5. W. S. Lee et al. "Age-Associated Decrease of Type IIA/B Human Skeletal Muscle Fibers." *Clinical Orthopaedics and Related Research* 450 (September 2006): 231–37.

6. Hwi Ryun Kwon et al. "Effects of Aerobic Exercise on Abdominal Fat, Thigh Muscle Mass and Muscle Strength in Type 2 Diabetic Subject." *Korean Diabetes Journal* 34, no. 1 (2010): 23–31.

7. E. G. Trapp et al. "The Effects of High-Intensity Intermittent Exercise Training on Fat Loss and Fasting Insulin Levels of Young Women." *International Journal of Obesity* 32 (2008): 24–28.

8. Westcott. "ACSM Strength Training Guidelines."

9. Trapp. "Effects of High-Intensity Intermittent Exercise Training."

10. A. Mourier et al. "Mobilization of Visceral Adipose Tissue Related to the Improvement in Insulin Sensitivity in Response to Physical Training in NIDDM: Effects of Branched-Chain Amino Acid Supplements." *Diabetes Care* 20, no. 3 (1997): 385–91.

11. Trapp. "Effects of High-Intensity Intermittent Exercise Training."

12. Jason L. Talanian et al. "Two Weeks of High-Intensity Aerobic Interval Training Increases the Capacity for Fat Oxidation during Exercise in Women." *Journal of Applied Physiology* 102, no. 4 (2007): 1439–47

13. Howard Hughes Medical Institute. "The Powerhouse—and Sentinal—of the Cell." May 31, 2006. http://www.hhmi.org/bulletin/may2006/features/mitochondria.html.

14. Howard Hughes Medical Institute. "Researchers Identify New Cause of Insulin Resistance." February 12, 2004. www.hhmi.org/news/shulman2.html.

15. Howard Hughes Medical Institute. "Cellular Power Plants Also Fend Off Viruses." August 26, 2005. www.hhmi.org/news/chen.html.

16. Talanian et al. "Two Weeks of High-Intensity Aerobic Interval Training."

17. Elizabeth V. Menshikova et al. "Effects of Exercise on Mitochondrial Content and Function in Aging Human Skeletal Muscle." *Journal of Gerontology* 61, no. 6 (2006): 534–40.

18. C. P. Earnest. "Exercise Interval Training: An Improved Stimulus for Improving the Physiology of Pre-Diabetes." *Medical Hypotheses* 71, no. 5 (2008): 752–61.

19. Stephen H. Boutcher. "Review Article: High-Intensity Intermittent Exercise and Fat Loss." *Journal of Obesity* 2011 (2011).

20. D. W. Lamson et al. "Mitochondrial Factors in the Pathogenesis of Diabetes: A Hypothesis for Treatment." *Alternative Medicine Review* 7 (April 2002): 94–111.

21. M. E. Patti et al. "The Role of Mitochondria in the Pathogenesis of Type 2 Diabetes." *Endocrinology Review* 31 (2010): 364–95.

22. F. G. Toledo et al. "Effects of Physical Activity and Weight Loss on Skeletal Muscle Mitochondria and Relationship with Glucose Control in Type 2 Diabetes." *Diabetes* 56 (2007): 2142–47.

23. David R. Broom et al. "The Influence of Resistance and Aerobic Exercise on Hunger, Circulating Levels of Acylated Ghrelin and Peptide YY in Healthy Males." *American Journal of Physiology—Regulatory Integrative and Comparative Physiology* 296, no. 1 (2008): R29–R35.

24. J. B. Li et al. "Effects of Exercise on the Levels of Peptide YY and Ghrelin." *Experimental and Clinical Endocrinology & Diabetes* 119, no. 3 (2011): 163–66.

25. Terry E. Jones et al. "Long-Term Exercise Training in Overweight Adolescents Improves Plasma Peptide YY and Resistin." *Obesity* 17, no. 6 (2009): 1189–95.

26. E. R. Ropelle et al. "IL-6 and IL-10 Anti-Inflammatory Activity Links Exercise to Hypothalamic Insulin and Leptin Sensitivity through IKKb and ER Stress Inhibition." *PLOS Biology* 8, no. 8 (2010): e1000465.

27. Mark Rakobowchuk et al. "Sprint Interval and Traditional Endurance Training Induce Similar Improvements in Peripheral Arterial Stiffness and Flow-Mediated ilation in Healthy Humans." *American Journal of Physiology—Regulatory, Integrative and Comparative Physiology* 295, no. 1 (2008): R236–42.

28. Trapp. "Effects of High-Intensity Intermittent Exercise Training."

29. W. L. Westcott and R. A. Winett. "Applying the ACSM Guidelines." *Fitness Management* 22, no. 1 (2006): 50Y4.

30. Charles Sturt University. "How Does Training Affect Performance?: Effect on Fast/Slow Twitch Muscle Fibres." http://www.hsc.csu.edu.au/pdhpe/core2/focus2/focus1/4007/2-1-4/fac2_1_4_6.htm.

31. Westcott. "ACSM Strength Training Guidelines."

32. C. Maria Kim et al. "Effects of Isokinetic Strength Training on Walking in Persons with Stroke: A Double-Blind Controlled Pilot Study." *Journal of Stroke and Cerebrovascular Dieases* 10, no. 6 (2001): 265–73.

33. J. W. Bea et al. "Resistance Training Predicts 6-Yr. Body Composition Change in Postmenopausal Women." *Medicine and Science in Sports and Exercise* 42, no. 7 (2010): 1286–95.

34. Westcott. "ACSM Strength Training Guidelines."

35. American Cancer Society. "Study Links More Time Spent Sitting to Higher Risk of Death: Risk Found to Be Independent of Physical Activity Level." http://pressroom.cancer.org/index.php?s=43&item=257.

36. Genevieve N. Healy et al. "Sedentary Time and Cardio-Metabolic Biomarkers in U.S. Adults: NHANES 2003–06." *European Heart Journal* 32 (2011): 590–97.

37. American Institute for Cancer Research: Science Now. "Breaking for Cancer Prevention." www.aicr.org/assets/docs/pdf/sciencenow/ScienceNow38-Fall-2011.pdf.

38. Marc T. Hamilton et al. "Too Little Exercise and Too Much Sitting: Inactivity Physiology and the Need for New Recommendations on Sedentary Behavior." *Current Cardiovascular Risk Reports* 2 (2008): 292–98.

39. Westcott. "ACSM Strength Training Guidelines."

40. Naomi Brooks et al. "Strength Training Improves Muscle Quality and Insulin Sensitivity in Hispanic Older Adults with Type 2 Diabetes." *International Journal of Medical Sciences* 4, no. 1 (2007): 19–27.

41. C. Pitsavos et al. "Resistance Exercise Plus to Aerobic Activities Is Associated with Better Lipids' Profile among Healthy Individuals: The ATTICA Study." *QJM: An International Journal of Medicine* 102, no. 9 (2009): 609–16.

42. W. L. Westcott et al. "Prescribing Physical Activity: Applying the ACSM Protocols for Exercise Type, Intensity, and Duration across 3 Training Frequencies." *Physician and Sportsmedicine* 2, no. 37 (2009): 51–58.

43. Washington State Department of Health. "What's the Big Deal about Controlling My Blood Pressure?" http://here.doh.wa.gov/materials/control-blood-pressure/13_BPbigPst_E12L.pdf.

44. K. Engelke et al. "Exercise Maintains Bone Density at Spine and Hip EFOPS: A 3-Year Longitudinal Study in Early Postmenopausal Women." *Osteoporosis International* 17, no. 1 (2006): 133–42.

Chapter 5. The 2-Day Diet Rules

1. L. T. Ho-Pham et al. "Veganism, Bone Mineral Density, and Body Composition: A Study in Buddhist Nuns." *Osteoporosis International* 20, no. 12 (2009): 2087–93.
2. H. R. Wyatt. "Long-Term Weight Loss and Breakfast in Subjects in the National Weight Control Registry." *Obesity Research* 10, no. 2 (2002): 78–82.
3. John M. de Castro. "The Time of Day of Food Intake Influences Overall Intake in Humans." *Journal of Nutrition* 134 (2004): 104–11.
4. US Food and Drug Administration. "Playing It Safe with Eggs." www.fda.gov/food/resourcesforyou/consumers/ucm077342.htm.
5. J. S. VanderWal. "Short-Term Effect of Eggs on Satiety in Overweight and Obese Subjects." *Journal of the American College of Nutrition* 24, no. 6 (2005): 510–15.

Chapter 6. Prep for Diet Success

1. A. M. Andrade. "Eating Slowly Led to Decreases in Energy Intake within Meals in Healthy Women." *Journal of the American Dietetic Association* 108, no. 7 (2008): 1186–89.
2. A. Kokkinos. "Eating Slowly Increases the Postprandial Response of the Anorexigenic Gut Hormones, Peptide YY and Glucagon-Like Peptide-1." *Journal of Clinical Endocrinology & Metabolism* 95, no. 1 (2010): 333–37.
3. University of Rhode Island. "URI Researcher Provides Further Evidence That Slow Eating Reduces Food Intake." Press release, October 27, 2011. http://www.uri.edu/news/releases/?id=6019. Also see Virginia Tech News. "Clinical Trial Confirms Effectiveness of Simple Appetite Control Method." Article, August 23, 2010. www.vtnews.vt.edu/articles/2010/08/082310-cals-davy.html.
4. Virginia Tech News. "Clinical Trial Confirms Effectiveness."
5. Vanderbilt University Medical Center. "Plain Water Has Surprising Impact on Blood Pressure." *Reporter*, July 8, 2010. www.mc.vanderbilt.edu/reporter/index.html?ID=9047.
6. C. M. Brown. "Water-Induced Thermogenesis Reconsidered: The Effects of Osmolality and Water Temperature on Energy Expenditure after

Drinking." *Journal of Clinical Endocrinology & Metabolism* 91, no. 9 (2006): 3598–602.

7. Christian Benedict. "Acute Sleep Deprivation Enhances the Brain's Response to Hedonic Food Stimuli: An fMRI Study." *Journal of Clinical Endocrinology & Metabolism* 97, no. 3 (2012): E443–47.

8. A. V. Nedeltcheva. "Insufficient Sleep Undermines Dietary Efforts to Reduce Adiposity." *Annals of Internal Medicine* 153, no. 7 (2010): 435–41.

9. M. L. Butryn. "Consistent Self-Monitoring of Weight: A Key Component of Successful Weight Loss Maintenance." *Obesity* 15, no. 12 (2007): 3091–96.

10. M. L. Kiem. "A Descriptive Study of Individuals Successful at Long-Term Maintenance of Substantial Weight Loss." *American Journal of Clinical Nutrition* 66, no. 2 (1997): 239–46.

11. C. G. Ulen. "Weight Regain Prevention." *Clinical Diabetes* 26 (July 2008): 100–13.

12. E. Newman. "Daily Hassles and Eating Behaviour: The Role of Cortisol Reactivity Status." *Psychoneuroendocrinology* 32, no. 2 (2007): 125–32.

13. G. Oliver. "Stress and Food Choice: A Laboratory Study." *Psychosomatic Medicine* 62, no. 6 (2000): 853–65.

14. G. Hawley. "Sustainability of Health and Lifestyle Improvements Following a Non-Dieting Randomised Trial in Overweight Women." *Preventive Medicine* 47, no. 6 (2008): 593–99.

15. J. Daubenmier. "Mindfulness Intervention for Stress Eating to Reduce Cortisol and Abdominal Fat among Overweight and Obese Women: An Exploratory Randomized Controlled Study." *Journal of Obesity* 2011 (2011).

Chapter 7. Phase 1: The 5-Day Jump Start

1. J. F. Hollis. "Weight Loss during the Intensive Intervention Phase of the Weight-Loss Maintenance Trial." *American Journal of Preventive Medicine* 35, no. 2 (2008): 118–26.

Chapter 8. Phase 2: The 2-Day Diet

1. R. De Weirdt. "Glycerol Supplementation Enhances *L. reuteri*'s Protective Effect against *S.* Typhimurium Colonization in a 3-D Model of Colonic Epithelium." *PLOS ONE* 7, no. 5 (2012).

2. R. Krajmalnik-Brown. "Effects of Gut Microbes on Nutrient Absorption and Energy Regulation." *Nutrition in Clinical Practice* 27, no. 2 (2012): 201.

3. J. A. Bravo. "Ingestion of Lactobacillus Strain Regulates Emotional Behavior and Central GABA Receptor Expression in a Mouse via the Vagus Nerve." *Proceedings of the National Academy of Sciences* 108, no. 38 (2011): 16050–55.

Chapter 10. Prep for Exercise Success

1. Prevention.com Expert Center. "Featured Question: When Is the Best Time of the Day to Exercise?" www.prevention.com/best-time-exercise#ixzz22Qj8kwKD.
2. J. T. Manire. "Diurnal Variation of Hamstring and Lumbar Flexibility." *Journal of Strength and Conditioning Research* 24, no. 6 (2010): 1464–71.
3. K. Van Proeyen. "Training in the Fasted State Improves Glucose Tolerance during Fat-Rich Diet." *Journal of Physiology* 588, pt. 21 (November 2010): 4289–302.
4. University of Dundee. "Study Finds Expensive Trainers a Waste of Money." Accessed October 11, 2012, www.prevention.com/best-time-exercise#ixzz22Qj8kwKD.

Chapter 12: After the Diet: Keeping the Weight Off

1. Harvie et al. "Intermittent Dietary Carbohydrate Restriction."
2. C. N. Sciamanna. "Practices Associated with Weight Loss versus Weight-Loss Maintenance: Results of a National Survey." *American Journal of Preventive Medicine* 41, no. 2 (2011): 159–66.
3. S. Byrne. "Weight Maintenance and Relapse in Obesity: A Qualitative Study." *International Journal of Obesity and Related Metabolic Disorders* 27, no. 8 (2003): 955–62.
4. S. Phelan. "Recovery from Relapse among Successful Weight Maintainers." *American Journal of Clinical Nutrition* 78 (2003): 1079–84.
5. www.sciencedaily.com/releases/2012/12/121210080511.htm.

APPENDIX A

Create Your Own Meals

Would you like to branch out and prepare dishes not included in the 2-Day Diet meal plan or in our easy-eating suggestions or mix-and-match lists? If you love to cook and want to work with other ingredients on the plan—or simply have a hankering for a food you haven't found in our recipe selection—you've come to the right place. In the next few pages, you'll find the carbohydrate and calorie counts (along with other nutritional information) for hundreds of foods, arranged by food group. (Carbs, fiber, net carbs, protein, and fat are provided in grams.)

FOOD	SERVING	CARBS	FIBER	NET CARBS	PROTEIN	FAT	CALORIES
Vegetables							
Artichokes:							
whole	1 medium	13.4	6.9	6.5	4.2	0.2	60
hearts, marinated	4	7	1	6	2	0	35
Asparagus	4 spears	2.6	1.2	1.4	1.5	0.2	25
Bamboo shoots	½ cup	2.1	0.9	1.2	1.1	0.3	12
Green beans	½ cup	5.3	2.1	3.2	1.3	2.2	41
Yellow wax beans	½ cup	4.9	2.1	2.9	1.2	0.2	22
Beets	½ cup	5.7	1.4	4.3	0.7	0.1	24
Bok choy	½ cup	0.8	0.4	0.4	0.5	0.1	4.5
Broccoli:							
raw	½ cup	2.4	0.9	1.5	1	0.1	12
cooked	½ cup	4.9	2.8	2.2	2.9	0.1	26
Broccoli rabe	½ cup	0.6	0.5	0.1	0.6	0.1	4.4
Brussels sprouts	½ cup	6.4	3.2	3.2	2.8	0.3	32
Cabbage:							
Chinese	½ cup	1.4	1.4	0	0.9	0.1	8
Green	½ cup	3.3	1.7	1.6	0.8	0.3	17
Red	½ cup	3.3	0.9	2.4	0.6	0.1	13.8
Savoy	½ cup	4.4	2.2	2.2	1.4	0.1	19.5
Carrots:							
sliced	½ cup	5.7	2.4	3.3	0.9	0.4	43
whole, 7½", raw	1	6.9	2	4.9	0.7	0.1	30
Cauliflower:							
raw	½ cup	2.6	1.3	1.4	1	0.1	13
steamed	½ cup	3.6	2.2	1.4	1.6	0.3	19
Celeriac	½ cup	4.6	0.9	3.6	0.7	0.2	21
Celery:							
cooked	½ cup	3	1.2	1.8	0.6	0.1	14
raw	1 stalk	1.2	0.6	0.6	0.3	0.1	6
Chard	½ cup	3	1.5	1.5	1.4	0.1	14
Collards	½ cup	4.1	2.4	1.7	1.8	0.3	22
Corn:							
on the cob	1 ear	14	1.8	12.2	2	0.5	58
cream style	½ cup	23.2	1.5	21.7	2.2	0.5	92
kernels	½ cup	14.7	2.1	12.6	2.5	0.9	66

FOOD	SERVING	CARBS	FIBER	NET CARBS	PROTEIN	FAT	CALORIES
Cucumber	½ cup	1.4	0.4	1	0.4	0.1	7
Dandelion greens	½ cup	3.4	1.5	1.9	1.1	0.3	17
Eggplant	½ cup	3.3	1.2	2.1	0.4	0.1	14
Endive	½ cup	0.8	0.8	0	0.3	0.1	4.2
Fava beans	½ cup	16.7	4.6	12.1	6.5	0.3	94
Fennel:							
cooked	½ cup	2.8	1.3	1.5	0.6	0.1	12
raw	½ cup	3.2	1.4	1.8	0.5	0.1	13
Garlic cloves	1	0.6	0.4	0.2	0.1	0	3
Jerusalem arti-choke	½ cup	13.1	1.2	11.9	1.5	0	57
Jicama, raw	½ cup	5.7	3.2	2.5	0.5	0.1	25
Kale	½ cup	3.6	1.3	2.3	1.2	0.3	18
Kohlrabi	½ cup	5.5	0.9	4.6	1.5	0.1	24
Lettuce:							
Boston/Bibb	½ cup	0.6	0.3	0.3	0.4	0.1	4
Iceberg	½ cup	0.8	0.4	0.4	0.3	0.1	4
Mixed greens	½ cup	1	0.5	0.5	0.4	0.1	5
Romaine	½ cup	0.7	0.5	0.2	0.5	0.1	4
Mushrooms:							
Portobello	4 oz	5.6	2.5	3.1	4.8	0.8	40
Shiitake, cooked	½ cup	10.4	1.5	8.8	1.1	0.2	40
Straw, canned	½ cup	4.2	2.3	1.9	3.5	0.6	29
Whole white, raw	½ cup	1.6	0.5	1.1	1.5	0.2 1	1
Mustard greens	½ cup	2.3	2.1	0.2	1.7	0.2	14
Okra	½ cup	4.7	2.4	2.3	1.8	0.2	23
Onions, raw	½ cup	7.5	1.4	6.1	0.9	0.1	32
Parsnips	½ cup	13.2	2.8	10.4	1	0.2	55
Snow peas	½ cup	5.6	2.2	3.4	2.6	0.2	34
Peas	½ cup	9.9	3	6.9	3.8	0.3	55
Peppers:							
Green, uncooked	½ cup	3.5	1.3	2.2	0.6	0.1	15
Red, uncooked	½ cup	4.5	1.6	2.9	0.7	0.2	19
Potatoes:							
baked	½ cup	14.7	1.5	13.2	1.7	1.6	78
boiled	½ cup	15.7	1.4	14.3	1.5	1.8	83

FOOD	SERVING	CARBS	FIBER	NET CARBS	PROTEIN	FAT	CALORIES
Radicchio	½ cup	0.9	0.2	0.7	0.3	0.1	5
Radishes	10	1.6	0.7	0.9	0.3	0.2	9
Rutabaga	½ cup	7.4	1.5	5.9	1.1	0.2	33
Sauerkraut	½ cup	3	2.1	0.9	0.7	0.1	14
Scallions	½ cup	3.7	1.3	2.4	0.9	0.1 1	6
Shallots	½ cup	13.4	0.6	12.9	2	0.1	58
Sorrel, cooked	½ cup	1.5	1.3	0.2	0.9	0.3 1	0
Spinach:							
frozen, steamed	½ cup	5.3	3.8	1.5	4.1	0.5	33
raw	½ cup	0.5	0.4	0.1	0.4	0.1	3
Squash, summer:							
raw	½ cup	1.9	0.6	1.3	0.7	0.1	9
cooked	½ cup	3.9	1.3	2.6	0.8	0.3	18
Squash, winter:							
Acorn, baked	½ cup	14.9	4.5	10.4	1.2	0.1	57
Butternut, baked	½ cup	10.8	3	10.8	0.9	0.1	41
Hubbard, boiled	½ cup	7.6	3.4	4.2	1.8	0.4	35
Pumpkin, boiled	½ cup	6	1.4	4.6	0.9	0.1 2	5
Pumpkin, canned	½ cup	9.9	3.5	6.4	1.3	2.2	58
Spaghetti, cooked	½ cup	5	1.1	3.9	0.5	0.2	21
Zucchini:							
raw	½ cup	1.9	0.8	1.1	0.8	0.1	9
steamed	½ cup	4	1.4	2.6	1.3	0.1	19
Sweet potatoes:							
baked, medium,	½ potato	11.8	1.9	9.9	1.1	0.1	51
boiled	½ cup	17.6	2.5	15.1	1.4	0.1	76
Tomatoes:							
Cherry	10	6.7	2	4.7	1.5	0.3	31
Plum	1	2.4	0.7	1.7	0.6	0.1	11
Small, fresh	1	3.6	1.1	2.5	0.8	0.2	16
Sun-dried, in oil	5 pieces	3.5	0.9	2.7	0.8	2.1	32
Turnip greens	½ cup	3.6	2.9	0.7	0.9	0.2 3	5
Turnips	½ cup	3.8	1.6	2.3	0.6	0.1	16
Water chestnuts	½ cup	9.7	2	7.7	0.7	0	40
Watercress	½ cup	0.2	0.2	0	0.4	0	2

FOOD	SERVING	CARBS	FIBER	NET CARBS	PROTEIN	FAT	CALORIES
Fruit							
Apple	½ medium	9.5	1.7	7.8	0.2	0.1	36
Applesauce:							
sweetened	½ cup	25.4	1.5	23.9	0.2	0.2	97
unsweetened	½ cup	13.8	1.5	12.3	0.2	0.1	52
Apricots:							
canned in juice	3 halves	13.3	1.7	11.6	0.7	0	52
dried	6 halves	13	1.9	11.1	0.8	0.1	50
fresh	3 whole	11.7	2.1	9.6	1.5	0.4	50
Avocado:							
Haas	½ cup	9.9	7.8	2.1	2.3	17.7	192
Florida	½ cup	9	6.4	2.6	2.6	11.6	138
Bananas	1 small	23.1	2.6	20.5	1	0.3	90
Blackberries:							
fresh	½ cup	6.9	3.8	3.1	1	0.4	31
frozen, sweetened,	½ cup	25.2	2.4	22.8	0.9	0.3	93
frozen, unsweetened	½ cup	11.8	3.8	8.1	0.9	0.3	48
Blueberries:							
fresh	½ cup	10.5	1.7	8.8	0.5	0.3	41
frozen sweetened	½ cup	25.2	2.4	22.8	0.5	0.2	93
frozen, unsweetened	½ cup	9.4	2.1	7.4	0.5	0.2	40
Boysenberries:							
fresh	½ cup	6.9	3.8	3.1	0.5	0.3	31
frozen, unsweetened	½ cup	8	3.5	4.5	0.7	0.2	33
Cherries:							
Sour, canned in water	½ cup	10.9	1.3	9.6	0.9	0.1	44
Sour, fresh	½ cup	6.3	0.8	5.5	0.5	0.2	26
Sweet, canned in water	½ cup	14.6	1.9	12.7	1	0.2	57
Sweet, fresh	½ cup	9.7	1.3	8.3	0.7	0.6	42
Cranberries, fresh	½ cup	6	2	4	0.2	0.1	23
Dates:							
dry, chopped	½ cup	62	6	56	1.8	0.4	240
fresh	3	18.3	1.9	6.4	0.5	0.1	68

FOOD	SERVING	CARBS	FIBER	NET CARBS	PROTEIN	FAT	CALORIES
Figs:							
canned, in water	½ cup	17.4	2.7	14.7	0.3	0.1	30
fresh	1 small	7.7	1.3	6.4	0.3	0.1	30
Fruit cocktail:							
canned, in heavy syrup	½ cup	23.5	1.2	22.2	0.5	0.1	91
canned, in water	½ cup	10.1	1.2	8.9	0.5	0.1	38
Gooseberries	½ cup	7.6	3.2	4.4	0.7	0.4	33
Grapefruit	½ cup	9.5	1.7	7.8	0.7	0.1	37
Grapes:							
Green, seedless	½ cup	14.2	0.8	13.4	0.5	0.5	57
Red, seedless	½ cup	14.2	0.8	13.4	0.3	0.2	57
Guava	½ cup	11.8	4.5	7.3	2.1	0.8	56
Kiwifruit	1	11.3	2.6	8.7	0.8	0.3	46
Kumquat	4	12.1	5	7.1	1.4	0.7	54
Lemon juice	2 Tbsp	2.6	0.1	2.5	0.1	0	8
Loganberries	½ cup	9.2	3.8	5.4	0.5	0.3	37
Mango:							
dried	1 piece	4.1	0.3	3.8	0.1	0.1	16
fresh	½ cup	14	1.5	12.5	0.4	0.2	54
Melons:							
Cantaloupe, cubes	½ cup	7.4	0.7	6.7	0.8	0.3	31
Cantaloupe	¼ melon	11.5	1.1	10.4	2.4	0.8	97
Crenshaw melon, cubes	½ cup	5.3	0.7	4.6	0.8	0.1	22
Honeydew, cubes	½ cup	7.8	0.5	7.3	0.4	0.1	30
Watermelon, cubes	½ cup	5.5	0.4	5.1	0.5	0.3	25
Nectarine	1 whole	14.3	2.3	12	1.4	0.4	60
Oranges:							
sections	½ cup	10.6	2.2	8.4	0.9	0.1	42
whole	1	16.3	3.4	12.9	1.4	0.1	64
Papaya:							
dried	1 piece	14.9	2.7	12.2	0.9	0.2	59
fresh, small	½ fruit	14.9	2.7	12.2	0.5	0.1	59
Passion fruit	¼ cup	13.8	6.1	7.7	1.3	0.4	57

FOOD	SERVING	CARBS	FIBER	NET CARBS	PROTEIN	FAT	CALORIES
Peaches:							
canned, in water	½ cup	7.5	1.6	5.9	0.5	0.1	29
dried	2 halves	16	2.1	13.8	0.9	0.2	62
fresh, small	1 whole	7.5	1.2	6.3	0.7	0.2	31
Pears:							
canned, in water	½ cup	9.5	2	7.6	0.2	0	35
Bartlett, fresh,	1 whole	25.1	4	21.1	0.7	0.7	98
Bosc, fresh	1 whole	21	3.3	17.7	0.5	0.6	82
Persimmon	½ cup	15.6	3	12.6	0.5	0.2	59
Pineapples:							
canned, in water	½ cup	10.2	1	9.2	0.5	0.1	39
fresh, chunks	½ cup	9.6	0.9	8.7	0.3	0.3	38
Plums:							
fresh	1 whole	3.7	0.4	3.3	0.2	0.2	16
canned, in water	½ cup	13.8	1.3	12.5	0.5	0	51
Pomegranate	¼ whole	6.6	0.2	6.4	0.4	0.1	26
Prunes:							
whole	4	21.1	2.4	18.7	0.9	0.2	80
canned, in heavy syrup	½ cup	32.6	4.5	28.1	1	0.2	123
Raisins:							
golden	1 Tbsp	8.2	0.4	7.8	0.4	0	31
seedless	1 Tbsp	8.1	0.7	7.4	0.3	0.1	31
Raspberries:							
fresh	½ cup	7.1	4.2	3	0.6	0.3	30
frozen, sweetened	½ cup	32.7	5.5	27.2	0.9	0.2	129
Rhubarb	½ cup	2.8	1.1	1.7	0.6	0.1	13
Strawberries:							
fresh	½ cup	5.5	1.4	4.1	0.5	2.3	24
frozen, sweetened	½ cup	33	2.4	30.6	0.7	0.2	122
frozen, unsweetened	½ cup	10.1	2.3	7.8	1.5	0.1	39
Tangerine	1 whole	9.3	1.3	8	0.6	0.2	37

FOOD	SERVING	CARBS	FIBER	NET CARBS	PROTEIN	FAT	CALORIES
Beans (Legumes)							
Black beans	½ cup	20.4	7.5	12.9	7.6	0.5	114
Black-eyed peas	½ cup	20.1	5.4	14.7	7.2	0.6	111
Chickpeas	½ cup	24.6	7.1	17.5	7.8	2.4	147
Great northern	½ cup	20	6	14	7	2	130
Kidney	½ cup	19.8	8.2	11.6	8.1	0.1	110
Lentils	½ cup	19.1	7.5	11.6	8.6	0.4	110
Lima beans	½ cup	21.2	7	14.2	7.3	0.4	115
Navy beans	½ cup	23.7	9.6	14.1	7.5	0.6	127
Split peas	½ cup	20.7	8.1	12.6	8.2	0.4	116
Pink beans	½ cup	23.6	4.5	19.1	7.7	0.4	126
Pinto	½ cup	21.9	7.4	14.6	7	0.4	117
Soybeans, green	½ cup	10	3.8	6.2	11.1	5.8	127
Tofu:							
Firm	½ cup	5.4	2.9	2.5	19.9	11	183
Regular	½ cup	2.3	0.4	2	10	5.9	94
Silken, firm	½ cup	2.7	0.1	2.6	7.8	3.1	70
Silken, soft	½ cup	3.2	0.1	3.1	5.4	3.1	62

FOOD	SERVING	CARBS	FIBER	NET CARBS	PROTEIN	FAT	CALORIES
Grains							
Barley, cooked	½ cup	22.2	3	19.2	0.8	0.4	97
Bran:							
Oat bran	2 Tbsp	3	0.7	2.3	0.8	0.2	10
Wheat bran	2 Tbsp	4.7	3.1	1.6	1.1	0.3	16
Bulgur, cooked	½ cup	16.9	4.1	12.8	2.8	0.2	76
Cornmeal	2 Tbsp	13.4	1.3	12.1	1.5	0.3	63
Kasha, cooked	½ cup	16.7	2.3	14.4	2.8	0.5	77
Millet, cooked	½ cup	20.6	1.1	19.5	1.1	0.1	104
Quinoa, dry	1¼ cups	29.3	2.5	26.8	5.6	2.5	159
Rice:							
Basmati, dry,	¼ cup	36	0	36	4	0	160
Brown, cooked	½ cup	22.4	1.8	20.6	1.5	0.9	108
Arborio, cooked	½ cup	26.7	0.9	25.8	2.2	0.2	121
White, cooked	½ cup	26.7	0	26.7	2.2	0.2	121
Wild, cooked	½ cup	17.5	1.5	16	3.3	0.3	83

FOOD	SERVING	CARBS	FIBER	NET CARBS	PROTEIN	FAT	CALORIES

Noodles and pasta (cooked):

FOOD	SERVING	CARBS	FIBER	NET CARBS	PROTEIN	FAT	CALORIES
Couscous, cooked	½ cup	18.2	1.1	17.1	3	0.1	88
Egg noodles, cooked	½ cup	19.9	0.9	19	2.8	12	106
Japanese somen	½ cup	24.2	1.4	22.8	3.5	0.2	115
Rice noodles	½ cup	21.9	0.9	21	0.8	0.2	96
Thai rice	½ cup	24.5	1	23.5	1.5	0.1	105
Udon (brown rice)	½ cup	19.6	1.6	18	4.1	1	103
Plain pasta, cooked	½ cup	19.5	3.4	16	1.8	0.5	88
Whole wheat	½ cup	27	3.3	23.7	4.6	1	100

Pasta from other grains (cooked):

FOOD	SERVING	CARBS	FIBER	NET CARBS	PROTEIN	FAT	CALORIES
Corn pasta	½ cup	22.5	3.1	19.4	2.1	0.1	100
Quinoa pasta	½ cup	17.5	1.2	16.3	2	1	90
Rice pasta	½ cup	21.8	0.3	21.5	2	0	105
Semolina pasta	½ cup	60.8	3.3	57.8	10.6	0.9	300
Spelt pasta	½ cup	20	2.5	17.5	4	0.8	95

Nuts and Nut Butters

Most of the fat in nuts is the good kind—monounsaturated fat and, in some cases, omega-3 fatty acids. These fats help your body process blood sugar, boost satisfaction, and help keep your heart and arteries healthy. We've included protein and calorie counts to help you plan meals on regular-carb days.

FOOD	SERVING	CARBS	FIBER	NET CARBS	PROTEIN	FAT	CALORIES
Almond butter	2 Tbsp	6.8	1.2	5.6	4.8	18.9	203
Almonds, slivered	2 Tbsp	3.3	1.6	1.7	3.5	8.6	102
Almonds, whole	24	5.7	3.4	2.3	6.1	14.6	166
Brazil nuts	7	3	2	1	4.1	18.8	186
Cashew butter	2 Tbsp	8.8	0.6	8.2	5.6	15.8	188
Cashews, whole	18	9	1	8	4	13	161
Chestnuts, roasted	6	30	2.9	27.1	1.8	1.2	138
Hazelnuts, whole	12	5	3	2	4	17	177
Macadamia butter	2 Tbsp	5	0	5	3	24	230
Macadamias, whole	12	4	2	2	2	21	203
Peanut butter	2 Tbsp	6.2	1.9	4.3	8.1	16.3	190
Peanuts, whole nuts	35	6	2	4	7	14	164
Pecans, whole	15	4	3	1	3	21	191
Pine nuts	2 Tbsp	2.4	0.8	1.7	4.1	8.6	96

FOOD	SERVING	CARBS	FIBER	NET CARBS	PROTEIN	FAT	CALORIES
Pistachio nuts, whole (no shells)	49	8	3	5	6	13	161
Pumpkin seeds, hulled	2 Tbsp	4.3	0.3	4	1.5	1.6	36
Sesame seeds	2 Tbsp	4.2	2.1	2.1	3.2	8.9	103
Soybeans, roasted,	¼ cup	9.5	5	4.5	10	7.2	133
Sunflower seeds, hulled	3 Tbsp	6.8	2.6	4.2	5.5	14.1	165
Sunflower seed butter	2 Tbsp	7	4	3	7	16	200
Walnut halves	14	4	2	2	4	18	185

Fats and Oils

FOOD	SERVING	CARBS	FIBER	NET CARBS	PROTEIN	FAT	CALORIES
Canola	1 Tbsp	0	0	0	0	14	124
Coconut	1 Tbsp	0	0	0	0	14	116
Corn	1 Tbsp	0	0	0	0	13.6	120
Olive	1 Tbsp	0	0	0	0	13.5	119
Peanut	1 Tbsp	0	0	0	0	13.5	119
Safflower	1 Tbsp	0	0	0	0	13.6	120
Sesame	1 Tbsp	0	0	0	0	13.6	120
Soybean	1 Tbsp	0	0	0	0	13.6	120

Dairy Products

Note: We've included fat grams for dairy products because even when the carbs are fairly low, full-fat dairy products can contain a lot of saturated fat. It's better, in terms of health and calories, to choose low-fat or fat-free milk and yogurt. You can also look for reduced-fat cheeses in the dairy case at the supermarket. Since there is no dietary fiber in plain dairy products, net carbs are the same as total carbs. We've also included protein, because some dairy products stand on their own as good sources of protein.

FOOD	SERVING	CARBS	FIBER	NET CARBS	PROTEIN	FAT	CALORIES
Buttermilk, 1% fat	1 cup	13	0	13	9	2.5	110
Cream:							
Half-and-half	1 Tbsp	0.6	0	0.6	0.4	1.7	20
Heavy cream	1 Tbsp	0.4	0	0.4	0.3	5.5	51
Whipped, heavy	2 Tbsp	0.4	0	0.4	0.3	5.5	52
Whipped, light	1 Tbsp	0.6	0	0.6	0.4	2.9	29
Nondairy creamer	1 Tbsp	2	0	2	0	1	20

FOOD	SERVING	CARBS	FIBER	NET CARBS	PROTEIN	FAT	CALORIES
Milk:							
Condensed	2 Tbsp	20.8	0	20.8	3	3.3	123
Evaporated, 2%	2 Tbsp	3.5	0	3.5	2.3	0.6	29
Evaporated, whole	2 Tbsp	3.2	0	3.2	2.2	2.4	42
Fat-free milk	1 cup	12.2	0	12.2	8.3	0.2	83
Low-fat, 1%	1 cup	12.2	0	12.2	8.2	2.4	102
Reduced-fat, 2%	1 cup	11.4	0	11.4	8.1	4.8	122
Whole	1 cup	13	0	13	8	8	146

Fish, Meat, and Poultry

FOOD	SERVING	CARBS	FIBER	NET CARBS	PROTEIN	FAT	CALORIES
Fish (cooked unless noted):							
Sea bass	6 oz	0	0	0	37.7	10	252
Striped bass	6 oz	0	0	0	38.7	5.1	211
Bluefish	6 oz	0	0	0	43.7	9.3	270
Catfish	6 oz	0	0	0	31	20	313
Cod	6 oz	0	0	0	35.6	6.1	208
Flounder	6 oz	0	0	0	37.4	7.2	225
Haddock	6 oz	0	0	0	38	6.3	218
Haddock, smoked	6 oz	0	0	0	42.9	1.6	197
Halibut	6 oz	0	0	0	45.4	5	238
Herring, in sour cream	1¼ cups	8	0	8	7	7	120
Mackerel	6 oz	0	0	0	38	23.5	377
Mahi mahi	6 oz	0	0	0	42	1.6	193
Perch	6 oz	0	0	0	42.3	2	199
Salmon:							
fresh, fillet	6 oz	0	0	0	40.8	13	291
canned	6 oz	0	0	0	35	10.7	245
smoked	6 oz	0	0	0	31.1	7.4	199
Sardines:							
canned, in mustard	6 oz	1.3	0	1.3	35.5	17.8	316
canned, in oil	6 oz	0	0	0	41.9	19.5	354
Scrod	6 oz	0	0	0	37.6	6.3	218
Shad	6 oz	0	0	0	26.9	30	429
Swordfish	6 oz	0.8	0	0.8	40.5	14	301
Trout	6 oz	0	0	0	41.5	15.6	319

FOOD	SERVING	CARBS	FIBER	NET CARBS	PROTEIN	FAT	CALORIES
Tuna	6 oz	0	0	0	46.4	6.7	259
White, canned, in oil	6 oz	0	0	0	45.1	13.7	316
White, canned, in water	6 oz	0	0	0	40.6	1.4	194
Shellfish:							
Clams	6 oz	5.5	0	5.5	27.2	2.1	157
Crab	6 oz	0	0	0	34.4	3	174
Crawfish	6 oz	0	0	0	25	1.6	122
Lobster	6 oz	2.2	0	2.2	34.9	1	167
Mussels	6 oz	12.6	0	12.6	40.5	7.6	293
Oysters	6 oz	5.9	0	5.9	10.6	3.7	104
Scallops	6 oz	4.9	0	4.9	34.7	6.7	228
Shrimp	6 oz	2.1	0	2.1	46.4	3.9	241
Squid	6 oz	6	0	6	32.2	8 2	36
Surimi	6 oz	17.4	0	17.4	20.5	2.2	174
Beef:							
Beef jerky stick	5 oz	1.1	0	0	3.2	2.5	39
Brisket	6 oz	0	0	0	44	41.7	563
Calf liver	6 oz	4.9	0	0	33.6	8.2	240
Chuck	6 oz	0	0	0	50.1	31.6	498
Eye round	6 oz	0	0	0	45.3	24	410
Ground chuck	6 oz	0	0	0	38.9	44	562
Ground round	6 oz	0	0	0	46.7	28.1	454
Prime rib	6 oz	0	0	0	37	56.4	667
Rib eye roast	6 oz	0	0	0	37	56.4	667
Roast	6 oz	0	0	0	38.7	45.6	576
Short ribs	6 oz	0	0	0	24	62	660
Sirloin steak	6 oz	0	0	0	34.2	21.6	344
Skirt steak	6 oz	0	0	0	35	13.8	276
Tenderloin	6 oz	0	0	0	37	11	258
Top loin	6 oz	0	0	0	51.7	12.3	332
Top sirloin	6 oz	0	0	0	34	21.6	342
Veal cutlet	6 oz	0	0	0	51.4	29.3	483
Lamb chops	6 oz	0	0	0	37.6	50.3	614
Leg of lamb	6 oz	0	0	0	48.1	13.2	325
Processed meats:							
Bacon	3 pieces	0.2	0	0.2	5.6	6.3	81
Canadian bacon	3 pieces	0.9	0	0.9	16.9	5.9	129

FOOD	SERVING	CARBS	FIBER	NET CARBS	PROTEIN	FAT	CALORIES
Processed meats: (cont.)							
Beef bologna	3 slices	2.3	0	2.3	6.4	10.3	129
Ham	6 oz	1.8	0	1.8	28.2	6.6	174
Liverwurst	6 oz	5.3	0	5.3	24.7	48.5	556
Pastrami	6 oz	0	0	0	37	9.9	248
Pepperoni	5 pieces	1.1	0	1.1	5.6	11.1	128
Beef hot dog	1	2.5	0	2.5	6.8	17.3	194
Salami	3 slices	0.8	0	0.8	5.3	9.3	110
Sausage:							
Breakfast sausage	1 link	0	0	0	7	7	90
Chorizo	2 oz	1.1	0	1.1	13.7	21.7	258
Kielbasa	2 oz	2.2	0	2.2	7.6	9.9	126
Pork and beef sausage	1 link	0.4	0	0.4	1.7	4.7	51
Pork sausage	1 piece	0.2	0	0.2	3.9	7.3	82
Pork:							
Chops:							
Center cut, bone in	6 oz	0	0	0	50.7	14.1	344
Loin chop, bone in	6 oz	0	0	0	37.3	43.3	549
Loin roast	6 oz	0	0	0	46.1	24.9	422
Pancetta	1 oz	0	0	0	12	16	200
Prosciutto	6 oz	0.5	0	0.5	47	14.2	331
Sausage, Italian	2 oz	2.4	0	2.4	10.7	15.3	192
Spare ribs	6 oz	0	0	0	31	32.6	427
Tenderloin	6 oz	0	0	0	47.9	8.2	279
Chicken:							
breast:							
skinless	6 oz	0	0	0	44	6.2	243
with skin	6 oz	0	0	0	50.7	13.2	335
drumstick:							
skinless	6 oz	0	0	0	48	15.8	348
with skin	6 oz	0	0	0	46	19	367
light and dark, meat only	6 oz	0	0	0	40.8	22.8	379
thigh, boneless, with skin	6 oz	0	0	0	42.6	26.4	420
Other poultry:							
Duck breast, no skin	6 oz	0	0	0	46.9	4.2	238
Turkey breast, no skin	6 oz	0	0	0	51.1	1.3	230

FOOD	SERVING	CARBS	FIBER	NET CARBS	PROTEIN	FAT	CALORIES
Turkey jerky	½ oz	1	0	1	9	0.5	50
Turkey sausage	2 oz	0.3	0	0.3	9.6	6.4	97

Sweeteners

FOOD	SERVING	CARBS	FIBER	NET CARBS	PROTEIN	FAT	CALORIES
Agave nectar	1 tsp	4	0	4	0	0	20
Brown rice syrup	1 tsp	5	0	5	0	0	20
Evaporated cane juice	1 tsp	4	0	4	0	0	15
Honey	1 tsp	5.5	0	5.5	0	0	21
Maple syrup	1 tsp	4.5	0	4.5	0	0	22
Molasses	1 tsp	4	0	4	0	0	16
Rapadura	1 tsp	4	0	4	0	0	15
Sucanat	1 tsp	4	0	4	0	0	15
Sugar, brown	1 tsp	4.5	0	4.5	0	0	17
Sugar, raw (turbinado)	1 tsp	5	0	5	0	0	20
Sugar, white	1 tsp	4	0	4	0	0	16

Noncaloric Sweeteners

Equal	1 packet	0	0	0	0	0	0
Splenda	1 packet	1	0	1	0	0	4
Stevia	1 packet	1	0	1	0	0	4
Sugar Twin	1 packet	0.5	0	0.5	0	0	0
Sweet'N Low	1 packet	less than 1	0	less than 1	0	0	0

Beverages

FOOD	SERVING	CARBS	FIBER	NET CARBS	PROTEIN	FAT	CALORIES
Beer:							
Regular beer	12 fl oz	12.8	0	12.8	1.7	0	154
Light beer	12 fl oz	0–5	0	0–5	0.7	0	99
Near beer	12 fl oz	5	0	5	1.1	0	32
Wine:							
Red	5 fl oz	2.7	0	4	0	0	88
White	5 fl oz	2.7	0	4	0	0	85
Wine cooler	5 fl oz	5.9	0	8	0.1	0	49
Hard liquor (all)	1 fl oz	0	0	0	0	0	82
Sherry, dry	3½ fl oz	1.4	0	1.4	0.2	0	72
Sherry, sweet	3½ fl oz	12.2	0	12.2	0.2	0	158

FOOD	SERVING	CARBS	FIBER	NET CARBS	PROTEIN	FAT	CALORIES
Tea:							
Brewed (black, green, white)	8 fl oz	0.7	0	0.7	0	0	2
Herbal, brewed	8 fl oz	0.5	0	0.5	0	0	2
Soda:							
Cola	12 fl oz	35.6	0	35.6	0	0	153
Diet soda	12 fl oz	0	0	0	0	0	0
Ginger ale	12 fl oz	31.8	0	31.8	0	0	124
Grape	12 fl oz	41.7	0	41.7	0	0	160
Lemon-lime	12 fl oz	38.3	0	38.3	0	0	147
Root beer	12 fl oz	39.2	0	39.2	0	0	152
Seltzer/club soda	12 fl oz	0	0	0	0	0	0
Fruit Juice:							
Apple	4 fl oz	14.5	0.1	14.4	4 0.1	0.1	58
Apricot	4 fl oz	18.1	0.8	17.3	0.5	0.1	70
Cranberry juice cocktail	4 fl oz	18.2	0.1	18.1	0	0.1	72
Grape	4 fl oz	18.9	0.1	18.8	0.7	0.1	77
Grapefruit, sweetened	13.9	4 fl oz	0.1	13.8	0.7	0.1	58
Grapefruit, unsweetened	4 fl oz	11.1	0.1	11	0.6	0.1	47
Guava	4 fl oz	19	1	18	0.2	0.1	74
Lemon	2 Tbsp	2	0.1	1.9	0.1	0	6
Lime	2 Tbsp	2.1	0.1	2	0.1	0	6
Mango 4 fl oz	18.9	0.9	18	0.3	0.1	73	
Orange	4 fl oz	12.9	0.3	12.6	0.9	0.3	56
Passion fruit	4 fl oz	16.8	0.2	16.6	0.5	0.1	63
Peach	4 fl oz	17.3	0.8	16.6	0.3	0	67
Pear	4 fl oz	19.7	0.8	18.9	0.1	0	75
Pineapple	4 fl oz	16	0.3	15.7	0.4	0.1	66
Prune	4 fl oz	22.3	1.3	21.1	0.8	0	91
Vegetable juice:							
Carrot	4 fl oz	11	1	10	0.9	0.2	47
Tomato	4 fl oz	5.2	0.5	4.7	0.9	0.1	21
Vegetable juice cocktail	4 fl oz	5.5	1	4.5	0.8	0.1	23

APPENDIX B

Keeping a Journal

What's your number one tool for continued success? Easy. It's keeping a food journal. A study from Kaiser Permanente's Center for Health Research, in which nearly 1,700 participants followed a health eating plan rich in fruits, veggies, and low-fat dairy, showed that people who kept daily food records lost twice as much weight as those who didn't. The simple act of writing down what you eat can make a huge difference in your weight-loss success.

We'll make it easy for you to get started. In the pages that follow, you'll find 2 weeks' worth of journal pages, where you can keep track of everything you eat as well as all your exercise routines. There's also room for you to note other important information, like how hungry you were before meals and how satisfied you felt afterward. Every now and then, you might want to look over your journal entries to see what made for a "good" day. (If you need more pages, feel free to photocopy these.)

Not a paper-and-pencil person? No problem! You can also track your eating on your computer or smart phone, on your desk calendar, or even on a sticky note. The most important thing: Just write it!

Journal Pages

FOOD DIARY

Today was a (check one): ___Low-Carb Day ___Regular-Carb Day

BREAKFAST

RATE YOUR HUNGER BEFORE EATING:	1 2 3 4 5 6 7 8 9 10
RATE YOUR SATISFACTION AFTERWARD:	1 2 3 4 5 6 7 8 9 10

LUNCH

RATE YOUR HUNGER BEFORE EATING:	1 2 3 4 5 6 7 8 9 10
RATE YOUR SATISFACTION AFTERWARD:	1 2 3 4 5 6 7 8 9 10

EXERCISE

☐ *INTERVAL WORKOUT* ☐ *TONING ROUTINE* ☐ *OTHER EXERCISE*

NOTES ABOUT YOUR EXERCISE TODAY:

Logging your meals, exercise, and experiences as you lose weight can lead to better results. Use these journal pages to start your own log. Copy if you need more.

DINNER

RATE YOUR HUNGER BEFORE EATING:	1	2	3	4	5	6	7	8	9	10
RATE YOUR SATISFACTION AFTERWARD:	1	2	3	4	5	6	7	8	9	10

SNACK

RATE YOUR HUNGER BEFORE EATING:	1	2	3	4	5	6	7	8	9	10
RATE YOUR SATISFACTION AFTERWARD:	1	2	3	4	5	6	7	8	9	10

PERSONAL NOTES

ENERGY LEVEL   1 2 3 4 5 6 7 8 9 10
(Circle one. 1 = "I'm so tired, I can barely move" and 10 = "I've got so much energy, I could dance all night!")

MOOD   1 2 3 4 5 6 7 8 9 10
(Circle one. 1 = "Down, low mood" and 10 = "I'm on top of the world!")

MENTAL FOCUS   1 2 3 4 5 6 7 8 9 10
(Circle one. 1 = "Serious brain fog, hard to concentrate" and 10 = "Mentally sharp, very focused")

SLEEP QUALITY   1 2 3 4 5 6 7 8 9 10
(Circle one. 1 = "I slept poorly" and 10 = "I slept great and woke refreshed and energized")

Journal Pages

FOOD DIARY

Today was a (check one): ___Low-Carb Day ___Regular-Carb Day

BREAKFAST

| RATE YOUR HUNGER BEFORE EATING: | 1 | 2 | 3 | 4 | 5 | 6 | 7 | 8 | 9 | 10 |
| RATE YOUR SATISFACTION AFTERWARD: | 1 | 2 | 3 | 4 | 5 | 6 | 7 | 8 | 9 | 10 |

LUNCH

| RATE YOUR HUNGER BEFORE EATING: | 1 | 2 | 3 | 4 | 5 | 6 | 7 | 8 | 9 | 10 |
| RATE YOUR SATISFACTION AFTERWARD: | 1 | 2 | 3 | 4 | 5 | 6 | 7 | 8 | 9 | 10 |

EXERCISE

☐ *INTERVAL WORKOUT* ☐ *TONING ROUTINE* ☐ *OTHER EXERCISE*

NOTES ABOUT YOUR EXERCISE TODAY:

Logging your meals, exercise, and experiences as you lose weight can lead to better results. Use these journal pages to start your own log. Copy if you need more.

DINNER

RATE YOUR HUNGER BEFORE EATING:	1	2	3	4	5	6	7	8	9	10
RATE YOUR SATISFACTION AFTERWARD:	1	2	3	4	5	6	7	8	9	10

SNACK

RATE YOUR HUNGER BEFORE EATING:	1	2	3	4	5	6	7	8	9	10
RATE YOUR SATISFACTION AFTERWARD:	1	2	3	4	5	6	7	8	9	10

PERSONAL NOTES

ENERGY LEVEL 1 2 3 4 5 6 7 8 9 10

(Circle one. 1 = "I'm so tired, I can barely move" and 10 = "I've got so much energy, I could dance all night!")

MOOD 1 2 3 4 5 6 7 8 9 10

(Circle one. 1 = "Down, low mood" and 10 = "I'm on top of the world!")

MENTAL FOCUS 1 2 3 4 5 6 7 8 9 10

(Circle one. 1 = "Serious brain fog, hard to concentrate" and 10 = "Mentally sharp, very focused")

SLEEP QUALITY 1 2 3 4 5 6 7 8 9 10

(Circle one. 1 = "I slept poorly" and 10 = "I slept great and woke refreshed and energized")

Journal Pages

FOOD DIARY
Today was a (check one): ___Low-Carb Day ___Regular-Carb Day

BREAKFAST

RATE YOUR HUNGER BEFORE EATING:	1	2	3	4	5	6	7	8	9	10
RATE YOUR SATISFACTION AFTERWARD:	1	2	3	4	5	6	7	8	9	10

LUNCH

RATE YOUR HUNGER BEFORE EATING:	1	2	3	4	5	6	7	8	9	10
RATE YOUR SATISFACTION AFTERWARD:	1	2	3	4	5	6	7	8	9	10

EXERCISE

☐ *INTERVAL WORKOUT* ☐ *TONING ROUTINE* ☐ *OTHER EXERCISE*

NOTES ABOUT YOUR EXERCISE TODAY:

TRACK YOUR SUCCESS!

Logging your meals, exercise, and experiences as you lose weight can lead to better results. Use these journal pages to start your own log. Copy if you need more.

DINNER

RATE YOUR HUNGER BEFORE EATING: 1 2 3 4 5 6 7 8 9 10
RATE YOUR SATISFACTION AFTERWARD: 1 2 3 4 5 6 7 8 9 10

SNACK

RATE YOUR HUNGER BEFORE EATING: 1 2 3 4 5 6 7 8 9 10
RATE YOUR SATISFACTION AFTERWARD: 1 2 3 4 5 6 7 8 9 10

PERSONAL NOTES

ENERGY LEVEL 1 2 3 4 5 6 7 8 9 10
(Circle one. 1 = "I'm so tired, I can barely move" and 10 = "I've got so much energy, I could dance all night!")

MOOD 1 2 3 4 5 6 7 8 9 10
(Circle one. 1 = "Down, low mood" and 10 = "I'm on top of the world!")

MENTAL FOCUS 1 2 3 4 5 6 7 8 9 10
(Circle one. 1 = "Serious brain fog, hard to concentrate" and 10 = "Mentally sharp, very focused")

SLEEP QUALITY 1 2 3 4 5 6 7 8 9 10
(Circle one. 1 = "I slept poorly" and 10 = "I slept great and woke refreshed and energized")

Journal Pages

FOOD DIARY

Today was a (check one): ___Low-Carb Day ___Regular-Carb Day

BREAKFAST

RATE YOUR HUNGER BEFORE EATING: 1 2 3 4 5 6 7 8 9 10

RATE YOUR SATISFACTION AFTERWARD: 1 2 3 4 5 6 7 8 9 10

LUNCH

RATE YOUR HUNGER BEFORE EATING: 1 2 3 4 5 6 7 8 9 10

RATE YOUR SATISFACTION AFTERWARD: 1 2 3 4 5 6 7 8 9 10

EXERCISE

☐ *INTERVAL WORKOUT* ☐ *TONING ROUTINE* ☐ *OTHER EXERCISE*

NOTES ABOUT YOUR EXERCISE TODAY:

Logging your meals, exercise, and experiences as you lose weight can lead to better results. Use these journal pages to start your own log. Copy if you need more.

DINNER

RATE YOUR HUNGER BEFORE EATING:	1 2 3 4 5 6 7 8 9 10
RATE YOUR SATISFACTION AFTERWARD:	1 2 3 4 5 6 7 8 9 10

SNACK

RATE YOUR HUNGER BEFORE EATING:	1 2 3 4 5 6 7 8 9 10
RATE YOUR SATISFACTION AFTERWARD:	1 2 3 4 5 6 7 8 9 10

PERSONAL NOTES

ENERGY LEVEL   1 2 3 4 5 6 7 8 9 10
(Circle one. 1 = "I'm so tired, I can barely move" and 10 = "I've got so much energy, I could dance all night!")

MOOD   1 2 3 4 5 6 7 8 9 10
(Circle one. 1 = "Down, low mood" and 10 = "I'm on top of the world!")

MENTAL FOCUS   1 2 3 4 5 6 7 8 9 10
(Circle one. 1 = "Serious brain fog, hard to concentrate" and 10 = "Mentally sharp, very focused")

SLEEP QUALITY   1 2 3 4 5 6 7 8 9 10
(Circle one. 1 = "I slept poorly" and 10 = "I slept great and woke refreshed and energized")

Journal Pages

FOOD DIARY

Today was a (check one): ___Low-Carb Day ___Regular-Carb Day

BREAKFAST

RATE YOUR HUNGER BEFORE EATING:	1	2	3	4	5	6	7	8	9	10
RATE YOUR SATISFACTION AFTERWARD:	1	2	3	4	5	6	7	8	9	10

LUNCH

RATE YOUR HUNGER BEFORE EATING:	1	2	3	4	5	6	7	8	9	10
RATE YOUR SATISFACTION AFTERWARD:	1	2	3	4	5	6	7	8	9	10

EXERCISE

☐ *INTERVAL WORKOUT* ☐ *TONING ROUTINE* ☐ *OTHER EXERCISE*

NOTES ABOUT YOUR EXERCISE TODAY:

TRACK YOUR SUCCESS!

Logging your meals, exercise, and experiences as you lose weight can lead to better results. Use these journal pages to start your own log. Copy if you need more.

DINNER

| RATE YOUR HUNGER BEFORE EATING: | 1 2 3 4 5 6 7 8 9 10 |
| RATE YOUR SATISFACTION AFTERWARD: | 1 2 3 4 5 6 7 8 9 10 |

SNACK

| RATE YOUR HUNGER BEFORE EATING: | 1 2 3 4 5 6 7 8 9 10 |
| RATE YOUR SATISFACTION AFTERWARD: | 1 2 3 4 5 6 7 8 9 10 |

PERSONAL NOTES

ENERGY LEVEL   1 2 3 4 5 6 7 8 9 10
(Circle one. 1 = "I'm so tired, I can barely move" and 10 = "I've got so much energy, I could dance all night!")

MOOD   1 2 3 4 5 6 7 8 9 10
(Circle one. 1 = "Down, low mood" and 10 = "I'm on top of the world!")

MENTAL FOCUS   1 2 3 4 5 6 7 8 9 10
(Circle one. 1 = "Serious brain fog, hard to concentrate" and 10 = "Mentally sharp, very focused")

SLEEP QUALITY   1 2 3 4 5 6 7 8 9 10
(Circle one. 1 = "I slept poorly" and 10 = "I slept great and woke refreshed and energized")

Journal Pages

FOOD DIARY

Today was a (check one): ___Low-Carb Day ___Regular-Carb Day

BREAKFAST

| RATE YOUR HUNGER BEFORE EATING: | 1 2 3 4 5 6 7 8 9 10 |
| RATE YOUR SATISFACTION AFTERWARD: | 1 2 3 4 5 6 7 8 9 10 |

LUNCH

| RATE YOUR HUNGER BEFORE EATING: | 1 2 3 4 5 6 7 8 9 10 |
| RATE YOUR SATISFACTION AFTERWARD: | 1 2 3 4 5 6 7 8 9 10 |

EXERCISE

☐ *INTERVAL WORKOUT* ☐ *TONING ROUTINE* ☐ *OTHER EXERCISE*

NOTES ABOUT YOUR EXERCISE TODAY:

TRACK YOUR SUCCESS!

Logging your meals, exercise, and experiences as you lose weight can lead to better results. Use these journal pages to start your own log. Copy if you need more.

DINNER

RATE YOUR HUNGER BEFORE EATING:	1	2	3	4	5	6	7	8	9	10
RATE YOUR SATISFACTION AFTERWARD:	1	2	3	4	5	6	7	8	9	10

SNACK

RATE YOUR HUNGER BEFORE EATING:	1	2	3	4	5	6	7	8	9	10
RATE YOUR SATISFACTION AFTERWARD:	1	2	3	4	5	6	7	8	9	10

PERSONAL NOTES

ENERGY LEVEL   1   2   3   4   5   6   7   8   9   10
(Circle one. 1 = "I'm so tired, I can barely move" and 10 = "I've got so much energy, I could dance all night!")

MOOD   1   2   3   4   5   6   7   8   9   10
(Circle one. 1 = "Down, low mood" and 10 = "I'm on top of the world!")

MENTAL FOCUS   1   2   3   4   5   6   7   8   9   10
(Circle one. 1 = "Serious brain fog, hard to concentrate" and 10 = "Mentally sharp, very focused")

SLEEP QUALITY   1   2   3   4   5   6   7   8   9   10
(Circle one. 1 = "I slept poorly" and 10 = "I slept great and woke refreshed and energized")

Journal Pages

FOOD DIARY

Today was a (check one): ___Low-Carb Day ___Regular-Carb Day

BREAKFAST

RATE YOUR HUNGER BEFORE EATING:	1 2 3 4 5 6 7 8 9 10
RATE YOUR SATISFACTION AFTERWARD:	1 2 3 4 5 6 7 8 9 10

LUNCH

RATE YOUR HUNGER BEFORE EATING:	1 2 3 4 5 6 7 8 9 10
RATE YOUR SATISFACTION AFTERWARD:	1 2 3 4 5 6 7 8 9 10

EXERCISE

☐ *INTERVAL WORKOUT*   ☐ *TONING ROUTINE*   ☐ *OTHER EXERCISE*

NOTES ABOUT YOUR EXERCISE TODAY:

Logging your meals, exercise, and experiences as you lose weight can lead to better results. Use these journal pages to start your own log. Copy if you need more.

DINNER

RATE YOUR HUNGER BEFORE EATING: 1   2   3   4   5   6   7   8   9   10
RATE YOUR SATISFACTION AFTERWARD: 1   2   3   4   5   6   7   8   9   10

SNACK

RATE YOUR HUNGER BEFORE EATING: 1   2   3   4   5   6   7   8   9   10
RATE YOUR SATISFACTION AFTERWARD: 1   2   3   4   5   6   7   8   9   10

PERSONAL NOTES

ENERGY LEVEL   1   2   3   4   5   6   7   8   9   10
(Circle one. 1 = "I'm so tired, I can barely move" and 10 = "I've got so much energy, I could dance all night!")

MOOD   1   2   3   4   5   6   7   8   9   10
(Circle one. 1 = "Down, low mood" and 10 = "I'm on top of the world!")

MENTAL FOCUS   1   2   3   4   5   6   7   8   9   10
(Circle one. 1 = "Serious brain fog, hard to concentrate" and 10 = "Mentally sharp, very focused")

SLEEP QUALITY   1   2   3   4   5   6   7   8   9   10
(Circle one. 1 = "I slept poorly" and 10 = "I slept great and woke refreshed and energized")

Journal Pages

FOOD DIARY

Today was a (check one): ___Low-Carb Day ___Regular-Carb Day

BREAKFAST

RATE YOUR HUNGER BEFORE EATING:	1 2 3 4 5 6 7 8 9 10
RATE YOUR SATISFACTION AFTERWARD:	1 2 3 4 5 6 7 8 9 10

LUNCH

RATE YOUR HUNGER BEFORE EATING:	1 2 3 4 5 6 7 8 9 10
RATE YOUR SATISFACTION AFTERWARD:	1 2 3 4 5 6 7 8 9 10

EXERCISE

☐ *INTERVAL WORKOUT* ☐ *TONING ROUTINE* ☐ *OTHER EXERCISE*

NOTES ABOUT YOUR EXERCISE TODAY:

Logging your meals, exercise, and experiences as you lose weight can lead to better results. Use these journal pages to start your own log. Copy if you need more.

DINNER

RATE YOUR HUNGER BEFORE EATING:	1	2	3	4	5	6	7	8	9	10
RATE YOUR SATISFACTION AFTERWARD:	1	2	3	4	5	6	7	8	9	10

SNACK

RATE YOUR HUNGER BEFORE EATING:	1	2	3	4	5	6	7	8	9	10
RATE YOUR SATISFACTION AFTERWARD:	1	2	3	4	5	6	7	8	9	10

PERSONAL NOTES

ENERGY LEVEL   1   2   3   4   5   6   7   8   9   10

(Circle one. 1 = "I'm so tired, I can barely move" and 10 = "I've got so much energy, I could dance all night!")

MOOD   1   2   3   4   5   6   7   8   9   10

(Circle one. 1 = "Down, low mood" and 10 = "I'm on top of the world!")

MENTAL FOCUS   1   2   3   4   5   6   7   8   9   10

(Circle one. 1 = "Serious brain fog, hard to concentrate" and 10 = "Mentally sharp, very focused")

SLEEP QUALITY   1   2   3   4   5   6   7   8   9   10

(Circle one. 1 = "I slept poorly" and 10 = "I slept great and woke refreshed and energized")

Journal Pages

FOOD DIARY

Today was a (check one): ___Low-Carb Day ___Regular-Carb Day

BREAKFAST

RATE YOUR HUNGER BEFORE EATING: 1 2 3 4 5 6 7 8 9 10

RATE YOUR SATISFACTION AFTERWARD: 1 2 3 4 5 6 7 8 9 10

LUNCH

RATE YOUR HUNGER BEFORE EATING: 1 2 3 4 5 6 7 8 9 10

RATE YOUR SATISFACTION AFTERWARD: 1 2 3 4 5 6 7 8 9 10

EXERCISE

☐ *INTERVAL WORKOUT*   ☐ *TONING ROUTINE*   ☐ *OTHER EXERCISE*

NOTES ABOUT YOUR EXERCISE TODAY:

TRACK YOUR SUCCESS!

Logging your meals, exercise, and experiences as you lose weight can lead to better results. Use these journal pages to start your own log. Copy if you need more.

DINNER

RATE YOUR HUNGER BEFORE EATING:	1 2 3 4 5 6 7 8 9 10
RATE YOUR SATISFACTION AFTERWARD:	1 2 3 4 5 6 7 8 9 10

SNACK

RATE YOUR HUNGER BEFORE EATING: 1 2 3 4 5 6 7 8 9 10

RATE YOUR SATISFACTION AFTERWARD: 1 2 3 4 5 6 7 8 9 10

PERSONAL NOTES

ENERGY LEVEL   1 2 3 4 5 6 7 8 9 10

(Circle one. 1 = "I'm so tired, I can barely move" and 10 = "I've got so much energy, I could dance all night!")

MOOD   1 2 3 4 5 6 7 8 9 10

(Circle one. 1 = "Down, low mood" and 10 = "I'm on top of the world!")

MENTAL FOCUS   1 2 3 4 5 6 7 8 9 10

(Circle one. 1 = "Serious brain fog, hard to concentrate" and 10 = "Mentally sharp, very focused")

SLEEP QUALITY   1 2 3 4 5 6 7 8 9 10

(Circle one. 1 = "I slept poorly" and 10 = "I slept great and woke refreshed and energized")

Journal Pages

FOOD DIARY

Today was a (check one): ___Low-Carb Day ___Regular-Carb Day

BREAKFAST

| RATE YOUR HUNGER BEFORE EATING: | 1 | 2 | 3 | 4 | 5 | 6 | 7 | 8 | 9 | 10 |
| RATE YOUR SATISFACTION AFTERWARD: | 1 | 2 | 3 | 4 | 5 | 6 | 7 | 8 | 9 | 10 |

LUNCH

| RATE YOUR HUNGER BEFORE EATING: | 1 | 2 | 3 | 4 | 5 | 6 | 7 | 8 | 9 | 10 |
| RATE YOUR SATISFACTION AFTERWARD: | 1 | 2 | 3 | 4 | 5 | 6 | 7 | 8 | 9 | 10 |

EXERCISE

☐ *INTERVAL WORKOUT* ☐ *TONING ROUTINE* ☐ *OTHER EXERCISE*

NOTES ABOUT YOUR EXERCISE TODAY:

TRACK YOUR SUCCESS!

Logging your meals, exercise, and experiences as you lose weight can lead to better results. Use these journal pages to start your own log. Copy if you need more.

DINNER

RATE YOUR HUNGER BEFORE EATING: 1   2   3   4   5   6   7   8   9   10
RATE YOUR SATISFACTION AFTERWARD: 1   2   3   4   5   6   7   8   9   10

SNACK

RATE YOUR HUNGER BEFORE EATING: 1   2   3   4   5   6   7   8   9   10
RATE YOUR SATISFACTION AFTERWARD: 1   2   3   4   5   6   7   8   9   10

PERSONAL NOTES

ENERGY LEVEL   1 2 3 4 5 6 7 8 9 10
(Circle one. 1 = "I'm so tired, I can barely move" and 10 = "I've got so much energy, I could dance all night!")

MOOD   1 2 3 4 5 6 7 8 9 10
(Circle one. 1 = "Down, low mood" and 10 = "I'm on top of the world!")

MENTAL FOCUS   1 2 3 4 5 6 7 8 9 10
(Circle one. 1 = "Serious brain fog, hard to concentrate" and 10 = "Mentally sharp, very focused")

SLEEP QUALITY   1 2 3 4 5 6 7 8 9 10
(Circle one. 1 = "I slept poorly" and 10 = "I slept great and woke refreshed and energized")

FOOD DIARY

Today was a (check one): ___Low-Carb Day ___Regular-Carb Day

BREAKFAST

RATE YOUR HUNGER BEFORE EATING:	1	2	3	4	5	6	7	8	9	10
RATE YOUR SATISFACTION AFTERWARD:	1	2	3	4	5	6	7	8	9	10

LUNCH

RATE YOUR HUNGER BEFORE EATING:	1	2	3	4	5	6	7	8	9	10
RATE YOUR SATISFACTION AFTERWARD:	1	2	3	4	5	6	7	8	9	10

EXERCISE

☐ *INTERVAL WORKOUT* ☐ *TONING ROUTINE* ☐ *OTHER EXERCISE*

NOTES ABOUT YOUR EXERCISE TODAY:

Logging your meals, exercise, and experiences as you lose weight can lead to better results. Use these journal pages to start your own log. Copy if you need more.

DINNER

| RATE YOUR HUNGER BEFORE EATING: | 1 2 3 4 5 6 7 8 9 10 |
| RATE YOUR SATISFACTION AFTERWARD: | 1 2 3 4 5 6 7 8 9 10 |

SNACK

| RATE YOUR HUNGER BEFORE EATING: | 1 2 3 4 5 6 7 8 9 10 |
| RATE YOUR SATISFACTION AFTERWARD: | 1 2 3 4 5 6 7 8 9 10 |

PERSONAL NOTES

ENERGY LEVEL   1 2 3 4 5 6 7 8 9 10

(Circle one. 1 = "I'm so tired, I can barely move" and 10 = "I've got so much energy, I could dance all night!")

MOOD   1 2 3 4 5 6 7 8 9 10

(Circle one. 1 = "Down, low mood" and 10 = "I'm on top of the world!")

MENTAL FOCUS   1 2 3 4 5 6 7 8 9 10

(Circle one. 1 = "Serious brain fog, hard to concentrate" and 10 = "Mentally sharp, very focused")

SLEEP QUALITY   1 2 3 4 5 6 7 8 9 10

(Circle one. 1 = "I slept poorly" and 10 = "I slept great and woke refreshed and energized")

Journal Pages

FOOD DIARY

Today was a (check one): ___Low-Carb Day ___Regular-Carb Day

BREAKFAST

RATE YOUR HUNGER BEFORE EATING:	1	2	3	4	5	6	7	8	9	10
RATE YOUR SATISFACTION AFTERWARD:	1	2	3	4	5	6	7	8	9	10

LUNCH

RATE YOUR HUNGER BEFORE EATING:	1	2	3	4	5	6	7	8	9	10
RATE YOUR SATISFACTION AFTERWARD:	1	2	3	4	5	6	7	8	9	10

EXERCISE

☐ *INTERVAL WORKOUT*　☐ *TONING ROUTINE*　☐ *OTHER EXERCISE*

NOTES ABOUT YOUR EXERCISE TODAY:

TRACK YOUR SUCCESS!

Logging your meals, exercise, and experiences as you lose weight can lead to better results. Use these journal pages to start your own log. Copy if you need more.

DINNER

RATE YOUR HUNGER BEFORE EATING:	1	2	3	4	5	6	7	8	9	10
RATE YOUR SATISFACTION AFTERWARD:	1	2	3	4	5	6	7	8	9	10

SNACK

RATE YOUR HUNGER BEFORE EATING:	1	2	3	4	5	6	7	8	9	10
RATE YOUR SATISFACTION AFTERWARD:	1	2	3	4	5	6	7	8	9	10

PERSONAL NOTES

ENERGY LEVEL　　　1　2　3　4　5　6　7　8　9　10
(Circle one. 1 = "I'm so tired, I can barely move" and 10 = "I've got so much energy, I could dance all night!")

MOOD　　　1　2　3　4　5　6　7　8　9　10
(Circle one. 1 = "Down, low mood" and 10 = "I'm on top of the world!")

MENTAL FOCUS　　　1　2　3　4　5　6　7　8　9　10
(Circle one. 1 = "Serious brain fog, hard to concentrate" and 10 = "Mentally sharp, very focused")

SLEEP QUALITY　　　1　2　3　4　5　6　7　8　9　10
(Circle one. 1 = "I slept poorly" and 10 = "I slept great and woke refreshed and energized")

Journal Pages

FOOD DIARY

Today was a (check one): ___Low-Carb Day ___Regular-Carb Day

BREAKFAST

RATE YOUR HUNGER BEFORE EATING:	1 2 3 4 5 6 7 8 9 10
RATE YOUR SATISFACTION AFTERWARD:	1 2 3 4 5 6 7 8 9 10

LUNCH

RATE YOUR HUNGER BEFORE EATING: 1 2 3 4 5 6 7 8 9 10
RATE YOUR SATISFACTION AFTERWARD: 1 2 3 4 5 6 7 8 9 10

EXERCISE

☐ *INTERVAL WORKOUT* ☐ *TONING ROUTINE* ☐ *OTHER EXERCISE*

NOTES ABOUT YOUR EXERCISE TODAY:

TRACK YOUR SUCCESS!

Logging your meals, exercise, and experiences as you lose weight can lead to better results. Use these journal pages to start your own log. Copy if you need more.

DINNER

| RATE YOUR HUNGER BEFORE EATING: | 1 | 2 | 3 | 4 | 5 | 6 | 7 | 8 | 9 | 10 |
| RATE YOUR SATISFACTION AFTERWARD: | 1 | 2 | 3 | 4 | 5 | 6 | 7 | 8 | 9 | 10 |

SNACK

| RATE YOUR HUNGER BEFORE EATING: | 1 | 2 | 3 | 4 | 5 | 6 | 7 | 8 | 9 | 10 |
| RATE YOUR SATISFACTION AFTERWARD: | 1 | 2 | 3 | 4 | 5 | 6 | 7 | 8 | 9 | 10 |

PERSONAL NOTES

ENERGY LEVEL   1 2 3 4 5 6 7 8 9 10
(Circle one. 1 = "I'm so tired, I can barely move" and 10 = "I've got so much energy, I could dance all night!")

MOOD   1 2 3 4 5 6 7 8 9 10
(Circle one. 1 = "Down, low mood" and 10 = "I'm on top of the world!")

MENTAL FOCUS   1 2 3 4 5 6 7 8 9 10
(Circle one. 1 = "Serious brain fog, hard to concentrate" and 10 = "Mentally sharp, very focused")

SLEEP QUALITY   1 2 3 4 5 6 7 8 9 10
(Circle one. 1 = "I slept poorly" and 10 = "I slept great and woke refreshed and energized")

Journal Pages

FOOD DIARY

Today was a (check one): ___Low-Carb Day ___Regular-Carb Day

BREAKFAST

RATE YOUR HUNGER BEFORE EATING:	1	2	3	4	5	6	7	8	9	10
RATE YOUR SATISFACTION AFTERWARD:	1	2	3	4	5	6	7	8	9	10

LUNCH

RATE YOUR HUNGER BEFORE EATING:	1	2	3	4	5	6	7	8	9	10
RATE YOUR SATISFACTION AFTERWARD:	1	2	3	4	5	6	7	8	9	10

EXERCISE

☐ *INTERVAL WORKOUT*   ☐ *TONING ROUTINE*   ☐ *OTHER EXERCISE*

NOTES ABOUT YOUR EXERCISE TODAY:

TRACK YOUR SUCCESS!

Logging your meals, exercise, and experiences as you lose weight can lead to better results. Use these journal pages to start your own log. Copy if you need more.

DINNER

RATE YOUR HUNGER BEFORE EATING:	1	2	3	4	5	6	7	8	9	10
RATE YOUR SATISFACTION AFTERWARD:	1	2	3	4	5	6	7	8	9	10

SNACK

RATE YOUR HUNGER BEFORE EATING:	1	2	3	4	5	6	7	8	9	10
RATE YOUR SATISFACTION AFTERWARD:	1	2	3	4	5	6	7	8	9	10

PERSONAL NOTES

ENERGY LEVEL   1 2 3 4 5 6 7 8 9 10
(Circle one. 1 = "I'm so tired, I can barely move" and 10 = "I've got so much energy, I could dance all night!")

MOOD   1 2 3 4 5 6 7 8 9 10
(Circle one. 1 = "Down, low mood" and 10 = "I'm on top of the world!")

MENTAL FOCUS   1 2 3 4 5 6 7 8 9 10
(Circle one. 1 = "Serious brain fog, hard to concentrate" and 10 = "Mentally sharp, very focused")

SLEEP QUALITY   1 2 3 4 5 6 7 8 9 10
(Circle one. 1 = "I slept poorly" and 10 = "I slept great and woke refreshed and energized")

Journal Pages

FOOD DIARY

Today was a (check one): ___Low-Carb Day ___Regular-Carb Day

BREAKFAST

| RATE YOUR HUNGER BEFORE EATING: | 1 2 3 4 5 6 7 8 9 10 |
| RATE YOUR SATISFACTION AFTERWARD: | 1 2 3 4 5 6 7 8 9 10 |

LUNCH

| RATE YOUR HUNGER BEFORE EATING: | 1 2 3 4 5 6 7 8 9 10 |
| RATE YOUR SATISFACTION AFTERWARD: | 1 2 3 4 5 6 7 8 9 10 |

EXERCISE

☐ *INTERVAL WORKOUT*   ☐ *TONING ROUTINE*   ☐ *OTHER EXERCISE*

NOTES ABOUT YOUR EXERCISE TODAY:

Logging your meals, exercise, and experiences as you lose weight can lead to better results. Use these journal pages to start your own log. Copy if you need more.

DINNER

| RATE YOUR HUNGER BEFORE EATING: | 1 2 3 4 5 6 7 8 9 10 |
| RATE YOUR SATISFACTION AFTERWARD: | 1 2 3 4 5 6 7 8 9 10 |

SNACK

| RATE YOUR HUNGER BEFORE EATING: | 1 2 3 4 5 6 7 8 9 10 |
| RATE YOUR SATISFACTION AFTERWARD: | 1 2 3 4 5 6 7 8 9 10 |

PERSONAL NOTES

ENERGY LEVEL   1 2 3 4 5 6 7 8 9 10
(Circle one. 1 = "I'm so tired, I can barely move" and 10 = "I've got so much energy, I could dance all night!")

MOOD   1 2 3 4 5 6 7 8 9 10
(Circle one. 1 = "Down, low mood" and 10 = "I'm on top of the world!")

MENTAL FOCUS   1 2 3 4 5 6 7 8 9 10
(Circle one. 1 = "Serious brain fog, hard to concentrate" and 10 = "Mentally sharp, very focused")

SLEEP QUALITY   1 2 3 4 5 6 7 8 9 10
(Circle one. 1 = "I slept poorly" and 10 = "I slept great and woke refreshed and energized")

Journal Pages

FOOD DIARY

Today was a (check one): ___Low-Carb Day ___Regular-Carb Day

BREAKFAST

| RATE YOUR HUNGER BEFORE EATING: | 1 2 3 4 5 6 7 8 9 10 |
| RATE YOUR SATISFACTION AFTERWARD: | 1 2 3 4 5 6 7 8 9 10 |

LUNCH

| RATE YOUR HUNGER BEFORE EATING: | 1 2 3 4 5 6 7 8 9 10 |
| RATE YOUR SATISFACTION AFTERWARD: | 1 2 3 4 5 6 7 8 9 10 |

EXERCISE

☐ *INTERVAL WORKOUT* ☐ *TONING ROUTINE* ☐ *OTHER EXERCISE*

NOTES ABOUT YOUR EXERCISE TODAY:

Logging your meals, exercise, and experiences as you lose weight can lead to better results. Use these journal pages to start your own log. Copy if you need more.

DINNER

RATE YOUR HUNGER BEFORE EATING:	1	2	3	4	5	6	7	8	9	10
RATE YOUR SATISFACTION AFTERWARD:	1	2	3	4	5	6	7	8	9	10

SNACK

RATE YOUR HUNGER BEFORE EATING:	1	2	3	4	5	6	7	8	9	10
RATE YOUR SATISFACTION AFTERWARD:	1	2	3	4	5	6	7	8	9	10

PERSONAL NOTES

ENERGY LEVEL   1 2 3 4 5 6 7 8 9 10
(Circle one. 1 = "I'm so tired, I can barely move" and 10 = "I've got so much energy, I could dance all night!")

MOOD   1 2 3 4 5 6 7 8 9 10
(Circle one. 1 = "Down, low mood" and 10 = "I'm on top of the world!")

MENTAL FOCUS   1 2 3 4 5 6 7 8 9 10
(Circle one. 1 = "Serious brain fog, hard to concentrate" and 10 = "Mentally sharp, very focused")

SLEEP QUALITY   1 2 3 4 5 6 7 8 9 10
(Circle one. 1 = "I slept poorly" and 10 = "I slept great and woke refreshed and energized")

Journal Pages

FOOD DIARY

Today was a (check one): ___Low-Carb Day ___Regular-Carb Day

BREAKFAST

| RATE YOUR HUNGER BEFORE EATING: | 1 2 3 4 5 6 7 8 9 10 |
| RATE YOUR SATISFACTION AFTERWARD: | 1 2 3 4 5 6 7 8 9 10 |

LUNCH

| RATE YOUR HUNGER BEFORE EATING: | 1 2 3 4 5 6 7 8 9 10 |
| RATE YOUR SATISFACTION AFTERWARD: | 1 2 3 4 5 6 7 8 9 10 |

EXERCISE

☐ *INTERVAL WORKOUT*   ☐ *TONING ROUTINE*   ☐ *OTHER EXERCISE*

NOTES ABOUT YOUR EXERCISE TODAY:

Logging your meals, exercise, and experiences as you lose weight can lead to better results. Use these journal pages to start your own log. Copy if you need more.

DINNER

RATE YOUR HUNGER BEFORE EATING:	1	2	3	4	5	6	7	8	9	10
RATE YOUR SATISFACTION AFTERWARD:	1	2	3	4	5	6	7	8	9	10

SNACK

RATE YOUR HUNGER BEFORE EATING:	1	2	3	4	5	6	7	8	9	10
RATE YOUR SATISFACTION AFTERWARD:	1	2	3	4	5	6	7	8	9	10

PERSONAL NOTES

ENERGY LEVEL   1   2   3   4   5   6   7   8   9   10

(Circle one. 1 = "I'm so tired, I can barely move" and 10 = "I've got so much energy, I could dance all night!")

MOOD   1   2   3   4   5   6   7   8   9   10

(Circle one. 1 = "Down, low mood" and 10 = "I'm on top of the world!")

MENTAL FOCUS   1   2   3   4   5   6   7   8   9   10

(Circle one. 1 = "Serious brain fog, hard to concentrate" and 10 = "Mentally sharp, very focused")

SLEEP QUALITY   1   2   3   4   5   6   7   8   9   10

(Circle one. 1 = "I slept poorly" and 10 = "I slept great and woke refreshed and energized")

Journal Pages

FOOD DIARY

Today was a (check one): ___Low-Carb Day ___Regular-Carb Day

BREAKFAST

RATE YOUR HUNGER BEFORE EATING:	1	2	3	4	5	6	7	8	9	10
RATE YOUR SATISFACTION AFTERWARD:	1	2	3	4	5	6	7	8	9	10

LUNCH

RATE YOUR HUNGER BEFORE EATING:	1	2	3	4	5	6	7	8	9	10
RATE YOUR SATISFACTION AFTERWARD:	1	2	3	4	5	6	7	8	9	10

EXERCISE

☐ *INTERVAL WORKOUT* ☐ *TONING ROUTINE* ☐ *OTHER EXERCISE*

NOTES ABOUT YOUR EXERCISE TODAY:

TRACK YOUR SUCCESS!

Logging your meals, exercise, and experiences as you lose weight can lead to better results. Use these journal pages to start your own log. Copy if you need more.

DINNER

RATE YOUR HUNGER BEFORE EATING: 1   2   3   4   5   6   7   8   9   10

RATE YOUR HUNGER BEFORE EATING: 1   2   3   4   5   6   7   8   9   10
RATE YOUR SATISFACTION AFTERWARD: 1   2   3   4   5   6   7   8   9   10

SNACK

RATE YOUR HUNGER BEFORE EATING: 1   2   3   4   5   6   7   8   9   10
RATE YOUR SATISFACTION AFTERWARD: 1   2   3   4   5   6   7   8   9   10

PERSONAL NOTES

ENERGY LEVEL   1   2   3   4   5   6   7   8   9   10
(Circle one. 1 = "I'm so tired, I can barely move" and 10 = "I've got so much energy, I could dance all night!")

MOOD   1   2   3   4   5   6   7   8   9   10
(Circle one. 1 = "Down, low mood" and 10 = "I'm on top of the world!")

MENTAL FOCUS   1   2   3   4   5   6   7   8   9   10
(Circle one. 1 = "Serious brain fog, hard to concentrate" and 10 = "Mentally sharp, very focused")

SLEEP QUALITY   1   2   3   4   5   6   7   8   9   10
(Circle one. 1 = "I slept poorly" and 10 = "I slept great and woke refreshed and energized")

Journal Pages

FOOD DIARY

Today was a (check one): ___Low-Carb Day ___Regular-Carb Day

BREAKFAST

| RATE YOUR HUNGER BEFORE EATING: | 1 | 2 | 3 | 4 | 5 | 6 | 7 | 8 | 9 | 10 |
| RATE YOUR SATISFACTION AFTERWARD: | 1 | 2 | 3 | 4 | 5 | 6 | 7 | 8 | 9 | 10 |

LUNCH

| RATE YOUR HUNGER BEFORE EATING: | 1 | 2 | 3 | 4 | 5 | 6 | 7 | 8 | 9 | 10 |
| RATE YOUR SATISFACTION AFTERWARD: | 1 | 2 | 3 | 4 | 5 | 6 | 7 | 8 | 9 | 10 |

EXERCISE

☐ *INTERVAL WORKOUT*　☐ *TONING ROUTINE*　☐ *OTHER EXERCISE*

NOTES ABOUT YOUR EXERCISE TODAY:

TRACK YOUR SUCCESS!

Logging your meals, exercise, and experiences as you lose weight can lead to better results. Use these journal pages to start your own log. Copy if you need more.

DINNER

RATE YOUR HUNGER BEFORE EATING: 1   2   3   4   5   6   7   8   9   10
RATE YOUR SATISFACTION AFTERWARD: 1   2   3   4   5   6   7   8   9   10

SNACK

RATE YOUR HUNGER BEFORE EATING: 1   2   3   4   5   6   7   8   9   10
RATE YOUR SATISFACTION AFTERWARD: 1   2   3   4   5   6   7   8   9   10

PERSONAL NOTES

ENERGY LEVEL   1   2   3   4   5   6   7   8   9   10
(Circle one. 1 = "I'm so tired, I can barely move" and 10 = "I've got so much energy, I could dance all night!")

MOOD   1   2   3   4   5   6   7   8   9   10
(Circle one. 1 = "Down, low mood" and 10 = "I'm on top of the world!")

MENTAL FOCUS   1   2   3   4   5   6   7   8   9   10
(Circle one. 1 = "Serious brain fog, hard to concentrate" and 10 = "Mentally sharp, very focused")

SLEEP QUALITY   1   2   3   4   5   6   7   8   9   10
(Circle one. 1 = "I slept poorly" and 10 = "I slept great and woke refreshed and energized")

Journal Pages

FOOD DIARY

Today was a (check one): ___Low-Carb Day ___Regular-Carb Day

BREAKFAST

| RATE YOUR HUNGER BEFORE EATING: | 1 | 2 | 3 | 4 | 5 | 6 | 7 | 8 | 9 | 10 |
| RATE YOUR SATISFACTION AFTERWARD: | 1 | 2 | 3 | 4 | 5 | 6 | 7 | 8 | 9 | 10 |

LUNCH

| RATE YOUR HUNGER BEFORE EATING: | 1 | 2 | 3 | 4 | 5 | 6 | 7 | 8 | 9 | 10 |
| RATE YOUR SATISFACTION AFTERWARD: | 1 | 2 | 3 | 4 | 5 | 6 | 7 | 8 | 9 | 10 |

EXERCISE

☐ *INTERVAL WORKOUT* ☐ *TONING ROUTINE* ☐ *OTHER EXERCISE*

NOTES ABOUT YOUR EXERCISE TODAY:

Logging your meals, exercise, and experiences as you lose weight can lead to better results. Use these journal pages to start your own log. Copy if you need more.

DINNER

RATE YOUR HUNGER BEFORE EATING: 1 2 3 4 5 6 7 8 9 10
RATE YOUR SATISFACTION AFTERWARD: 1 2 3 4 5 6 7 8 9 10

SNACK

RATE YOUR HUNGER BEFORE EATING: 1 2 3 4 5 6 7 8 9 10
RATE YOUR SATISFACTION AFTERWARD: 1 2 3 4 5 6 7 8 9 10

PERSONAL NOTES

ENERGY LEVEL   1 2 3 4 5 6 7 8 9 10
(Circle one. 1 = "I'm so tired, I can barely move" and 10 = "I've got so much energy, I could dance all night!")

MOOD   1 2 3 4 5 6 7 8 9 10
(Circle one. 1 = "Down, low mood" and 10 = "I'm on top of the world!")

MENTAL FOCUS   1 2 3 4 5 6 7 8 9 10
(Circle one. 1 = "Serious brain fog, hard to concentrate" and 10 = "Mentally sharp, very focused")

SLEEP QUALITY   1 2 3 4 5 6 7 8 9 10
(Circle one. 1 = "I slept poorly" and 10 = "I slept great and woke refreshed and energized")

Journal Pages

FOOD DIARY

Today was a (check one): ___Low-Carb Day ___Regular-Carb Day

BREAKFAST

RATE YOUR HUNGER BEFORE EATING:	1	2	3	4	5	6	7	8	9	10
RATE YOUR SATISFACTION AFTERWARD:	1	2	3	4	5	6	7	8	9	10

LUNCH

RATE YOUR HUNGER BEFORE EATING:	1	2	3	4	5	6	7	8	9	10
RATE YOUR SATISFACTION AFTERWARD:	1	2	3	4	5	6	7	8	9	10

EXERCISE

☐ *INTERVAL WORKOUT* ☐ *TONING ROUTINE* ☐ *OTHER EXERCISE*

NOTES ABOUT YOUR EXERCISE TODAY:

Logging your meals, exercise, and experiences as you lose weight can lead to better results. Use these journal pages to start your own log. Copy if you need more.

DINNER

| RATE YOUR HUNGER BEFORE EATING: | 1 2 3 4 5 6 7 8 9 10 |
| RATE YOUR SATISFACTION AFTERWARD: | 1 2 3 4 5 6 7 8 9 10 |

SNACK

| RATE YOUR HUNGER BEFORE EATING: | 1 2 3 4 5 6 7 8 9 10 |
| RATE YOUR SATISFACTION AFTERWARD: | 1 2 3 4 5 6 7 8 9 10 |

PERSONAL NOTES

ENERGY LEVEL　　　1 2 3 4 5 6 7 8 9 10
(Circle one. 1 = "I'm so tired, I can barely move" and 10 = "I've got so much energy, I could dance all night!")

MOOD　　　1 2 3 4 5 6 7 8 9 10
(Circle one. 1 = "Down, low mood" and 10 = "I'm on top of the world!")

MENTAL FOCUS　　　1 2 3 4 5 6 7 8 9 10
(Circle one. 1 = "Serious brain fog, hard to concentrate" and 10 = "Mentally sharp, very focused")

SLEEP QUALITY　　　1 2 3 4 5 6 7 8 9 10
(Circle one. 1 = "I slept poorly" and 10 = "I slept great and woke refreshed and energized")

INDEX

Boldface page references indicate illustrations. <u>Underscored</u> references indicate tables or boxed text.